Therapy
For Young Stutterers

Therapy
For Young Stutterers
The Kopp Method

by Elwood G. Anderson

A Savoyard Book

Detroit Wayne State University Press 1970

Revised Edition
Published simultaneously in Canada
by The Copp Clark Publishing Company
517 Wellington Street, West
Toronto 2B, Canada.

Library of Congress Catalog Card Number: 74-96726
Standard Book Number: 8143-1413-4

Dedicated to the memory of
George Adams Kopp,
Professor, Therapist, Mentor, and Counselor

Contents

Preface

This handbook outlines a therapy for the treatment of stuttering based on the Organismic Method. It is geared to the level of the preschool and early elementary school child, grades kindergarten through 3A.

The Organismic or Kopp Method for the correction of a stuttering disorder can be found in Kopp's *Syllabus for Speech Correction.** This publication treats diagnostic as well as the therapy procedures. Another relevant publication is Elise Hahn's *Significant Theories and Therapies,*** which carries a summary statement of the method. Also, my doctoral dissertation, on file at the Wayne State University Library, discusses the Kopp Method and therapy.

I was severely handicapped with the disorder of stuttering from the elementary grades through undergraduate college. Earlier treatment at a well-known and established clinic in the State of Michigan produced no improvement.

In 1952, while I was a graduate student at Wayne State University, Dr. George A. Kopp, then director of the Speech and Hearing Clinic, provided me with the therapy necessary to overcome the disorder. Needless to say, I am eternally grateful to Dr. Kopp.

Since 1954, I have been a speech therapist.

E.G.A.

*(Ann Arbor, 1946).
**(Stanford, 1958), p. 71.

Introduction

The miracle of speech is a prime characteristic and evolutionary attribute of man alone. It separates him from the atavistic world. Speech has been man's most powerful weapon in his attempt to conquer the universe and thus to create an artificial environment. It gives man the power to interact within his society. Speech has given man the tool to forge a better society within a concurring governmental system. His endowment allows him the privilege of eloquent expression.

Those without speech fluency are disabled. One group of the speech handicapped are stutterers, who represent one of the largest groups of all speech handicapped persons.

Few issues in speech correction, pathology, and science have aroused as much controversy as stuttering theories and therapies, and the debate takes place not only among workers in the profession, but with psychologists and others as well. The problem of stuttering is important by virtue of the nature of the disorder, its implications for intelligent therapy, the effects of the problem on the possessor, and the number of persons afflicted.

The stutterer seeks relief from stuttering because he has a will to proclaim and an ego to satisfy. For the stutterer, relaxing mentally in society is not possible; he can only exist. And this is insufficient to ensure happiness. He seeks a form of existence that allows him the freedom to pursue a course of excellence, the power to create, invent, and set standards. He needs to dissipate barriers toward goals that make him unique in his conquest of life-space, where the powers of nature are subdued. The stutterer hopes that his body and mind can be trained to become the ready servants of his will and to do with pleasure all the work that he is capable of doing.

It is estimated that there are more than one million, stutterers in the United States, or seven individuals in every thousand.[1] However, in the majority of cases, the treatment of stuttering has not given the possessor the anticipated remediation. The stutterer and treatment, taken as a whole, is described by Lowenfeld:[2]

> Authorities agree . . . that stuttering is purely psychological in origin—a problem of emotional maladjustment involving the total personality. While the cause of stuttering is clearly psychological, there is no doubt that it results in a disturbance of motor coordination, that is, the inability to control those organs responsible for producing speech.

Current therapies reflect this assumed causality; and the speech practices for the correction of stuttering, Kopp Method excepted, are psychologically oriented, and the speech therapist allocates the major portion of the therapeutic session to life adjustment, relaxation, and parental counseling. Yet, this methodology has produced relatively little success.

Methods of therapy, like degrees of ability, vary, but the standard to use in the assessment of therapy is success. Success with Kopp therapy is evident with speech procedures applicable to the young, old, male, female, individual, or group, with little economic output.

Stuttering therapy dates back to Moses and the ancient Egyptians. Herodotus (484–424 B.C.), the Greek historian, records the treatment of Battos, son of Polymnestos, by a Pythian priestess. Hippocrates (760–370 B.C.), the "Father of Medicine," administered healing oils which, however, usually resulted in suppurated ulcers. Aristotle (384–322 B.C.) theorized about the disorder and recommended mirror-watching for treatment. Demosthenes (383–322 B.C.) overcame his stuttering by practicing declamations while walking uphill with pebbles in his mouth. Celsus (42 B.C.–A.D. 37) practiced breathing exercises, and Galen (A.D. 131–201) felt that cauterization of the tongue was necessary to correct the problem.[3] The early twentieth century produced concepts by Freud and Coriat, and interpretations of Scripture in which stuttering of words was regarded as related to psychic shocks, or concealed sexual and obscene thoughts, or infantile oral eroticism. Otto Fenichel believed stuttering to be a pregenital conversion neurosis. The result was a conflict between antagonistic tendencies. The stutterer wishes to say something, and yet does not say it for some unconscious reason.

In 1958, six authorities on stuttering summarized ideas about causes of the problem.[4] Oliver Bloodstein considered stuttering to be an anticipatory struggle reaction. Peter Glauber favored a psychoanalytic approach. Joseph Sheehan considered the problem to be one of conflict in terms of speaking and holding back of speaking, thus causing a conflict and avoidance problem. Robert West viewed the problem from an "agnostic" approach. Charles VanRiper held that stuttering was probably of a multiple origin, but that the important factor was the inability to perform linguistic tasks at the norm level; and Jon Eisenson believed that stuttering was the result of perseveration.

A different approach to an old problem is needed—one that treats the disorder on Gestalt principles and one that replaces abnormal speech patterns with normal ones. This method of treatment for stuttering is called the Organismic, or Kopp, Method.

The method, developed by Dr. George Kopp while he was at Columbia University in 1940, combines many years of research in all areas of the human organism in designing a new therapy for stuttering. This method has produced excellent results in both individual and group therapy. It is the only therapy which advocates the complete synthesis of cognitive-motor output for the correction of stuttering speech patterns.

The Kopp approach and philosophy, when compared with other therapies, shows a distinct difference and includes the following concepts:[5]

1) It considers the entire speech mechanism and the corresponding elements of speech and sound that are integrated in the total act of speaking.
2) It is based on the fact that language acquisition is additive in nature. Regressions in use of language verify this concept, which was established by research.
3) Because speech is produced from many cognitive-motor patterns, the goal of training is to replace the cognitive-motor pattern of stuttering with a cognitive-motor pattern of normal speech.
4) The cognitive-motor pattern of stuttering remains in the memory bank and may be recalled and used under certain conditions.
5) The Organismic Method differs from other methods in that it does not attempt to condition or modify the existing cognitive-motor pattern of stuttering. It does not reinforce abnormal speech habits.
6) Training involves exercises for the various muscles groups used in speech to establish range, strength, accuracy, and rate of function within the potential of the individual stutterer.
7) Controls of the new normal cognitive-motor patterns are established by minimizing interfering central activity and by establishing a monitoring system of respiration, phonation, resonation, and articulation through auditory and motor feedbacks.
8) Automaticity of normal function is effected by using established controls in various speaking situations.
9) The Organismic Method emphasizes the normal development of speech in all of its parameters.

Specifically, the method synthesizes psychomotor (cognitive-motor) functions for the practical elimination of spasmophemic conditions. This therapy includes the total input and output processes and begins with the examination and evaluation of the speaker.

Remedial procedures are carried out in the treatment areas of respiration, phonation, resonation, articulation, and cerebration.

The therapy begins with the area of respiration. Breathing

is the primary requisite for phonation, because normal voicings cannot be produced without air. The action of the respiratory process alters the volume of the chest cavity to create a ballistic impulse for the syllabic utterance. Therefore, the overall breath patterns must be corrected for normal breath support and control in stuttering therapy.

Phonation, the second area of treatment, is a function of the larynx. Therapy here seeks to produce smooth vocal attacks, which are the audible effect of vocal cord positioning in initiating the phonic action, and to produce precise and appropriate movements with respective subglottal pressure by establishing normal patterns in the use of the intrinsic and extrinsic muscles of the larynx.

Resonation, the third area of treatment, is the basis of voice quality, which is an identifying characteristic of each human voice. In resonation, there is an alteration of the coupled cavities to amplify or dampen band frequencies during shaping of the oral tract. Every change of pitch, vowel, or vowel color demands a special adjustment of the cavities.

Articulation, which functions as an integral part of the previous treatment, is the fourth area of treatment. It is concerned with functional efficiency of the tongue, lips, and jaw as affecting the range, strength, rate, and accuracy of the sound being produced.

Cerebration, the final treatment area, is equal in importance to those previously mentioned. Cerebration trains the mind of the stutterer for the purpose of closing the psychomotor loop for normal oral productivity.

The Kopp system works on the premise that it is of little value to try and talk stutterers out of their obsessions, delusions, opinions, and prejudices because they were acquired under experiential conditions. Thus, it is an environment which has its modus operandi in the thalamus. It fully recognizes that the thalamus cannot understand the theoretical symbolic orientations of language any more than a child can comprehend the nature of the universe. However, the use of the Kopp Method has yielded outstanding results at all age levels, especially with the preschool and elementary age group. It is possible to provide this therapy to children and adults in a combined therapeutic setting without loss of efficiency.

Finally, the philosophy underlying the method relegates fear, anxiety, and other components of emotion to secondary importance because experience has taught that they are related to the stuttering act as an outcome of the disorder through growth and the additive nature of language. Therefore, they are considered as a symptom; they are not construed as the primary cause in the majority of stuttering cases.

Rapport and Motivation

Rapport between therapist and parents is as necessary for this treatment as is rapport with the child. Thus, if the speech problem is related to parental behavior, home environment, health, or security, the elimination of the tension or stuttering-causing conditions can be accomplished.

Proper parental attitudes are essential to successful therapy. Parents can aid their child's progress by:[6] 1) becoming as sensitive as possible to the child's many ways of communicating, both verbally and nonverbally; 2) understanding the feelings being expressed as well as the intellectual content spoken; 3) providing a good speech model and making sentences of normal length; 4) listening to the child when he speaks and being interested in the message; 5) not expecting too much from the child and keeping the speech demands geared to his age and I.Q. level; 6) motivating the child through love and not hate (this will prevent harm to his ego development); 7) encouraging self-expression as often as possible; 8) never labeling the child as a stutterer; 9) spending a reading period with the child and speaking slowly enough so that he can follow every word; 10) giving the child things he can do and being generous with praise for even small successes; 11) giving the child adequate health protection; 12) assuring the child that the parent has planned for his happiness and security.

The goals of these procedures are to remove or overcome any form of anxiety, fear, feeling of insecurity, or health problems which may aggravate the disorder, and to create an atmosphere of quietness and freedom from tension and competition for a period of time sufficient to lay a new speech and reaction pattern. If these goals can be accomplished soon after the onset of the stuttering patterns in the child, he may return to normal speech habits without extensive therapy. This is especially true if fluent speech patterns were established prior to stuttering.

Therapy

All phases in the following therapy must first be practiced on a conscious level to establish the desired motor skills necessary to produce normal speech patterns. As these new skills are learned and maintained, the child can gradually structure them to involve the total speaking mechanism. The objective is to have all speech activity function automatically and without interference to stimuli requiring oral communication.

The therapist must have a working knowledge of the physiological bases of the practices presented here. In addition, the worker must be aware of normal as well as abnormal muscle movements.

In respiration, a common fault in stutterers is the failure to coordinate the breathing mechanism for speech. Consequently, the goal of therapy is the production of coordinated movements of breathing patterns for loudness or volume and smoothness of exhalation.

Phonation exercises attempt to correct the monopitch, which is usually present in stutterers. A variation of vocal tone is needed to convey mood and word connotation and to produce proper inflectional patterns.

The resonation practices are intended to alter the size, shape, and position of the resonating cavities through which the breath stream is directed. Cavity coupling is essential if the stutterer is to achieve good vocal quality and relaxed tones.

The section on articulation provides the basic exercises for improving the range, rate, strength, and accuracy of articulatory movements, which are necessary for the complex coordination of speech.[7] All movements must be smooth, relaxed, and rapid enough for the text involved.

The section on cerebration deals with the psychological aspects of training the stutterer to use his newly acquired skills in all speaking situations with ease and confidence.

Total mastery of each exercise in each unit is a prerequisite for the one that follows.

The materials necessary for the effective use of this manual include a chalkboard and accessories, tongue blades, tape recorder with tape loop, record player with selections including sound effects, animal noises, recorded messages, musical arrangements, and a complete book of nursery rhymes.

Respiration

The major goal of this unit is the establishment of correct breathing patterns for all forms of oral activity with regard to smoothness of function and volume. The child should be able to vary the loudness levels at least throughout a long sentence.

Various breathing patterns can be utilized in the speaking process—thoracic, diaphragmatic, abdominal, costal, and combinations of these types. For the stuttering child the easiest correctional pattern to learn and control is the diaphragmatic-abdominal combination. This approach closely resembles quiet breathing and the breathing patterns of sleep.[8]

Exercises for the controlled breathing patterns required for the process of speaking must be done consciously; and they must be practiced for intervals sufficient to accomplish specific goals.

The specific goals of the exercises are the ability to: 1) fill the lungs to their capacity either quickly or slowly; 2) exhale as quickly or as slowly as the occasion demands; 3) stop inspiration or expiration and resume the process at will without losing any of the already inspired breath; 4) phonate and sustain a pure vowel on exhalation for periods of twenty to twenty-five seconds (example: ō); 5) breathe quietly; 6) breathe so that the fullest inspiration brings no fatigue or physiological apnea; 7) economize the breath stream so that the supply is never exhausted; 8) economize the air stream during phonation; 9) breathe so naturally that neither breath nor the lack of breath is noticed by the listener; 10) vary the loudness at will with respect to meaning and to produce smooth exhalation patterns. These exercises for respiration have been very successful with all stutterers treated thus far at the Wayne State University Speech and Hearing Clinic and in the Detroit Public Schools.

The therapist should instruct the child by placing one hand on the diaphragm with the thumb at the base of the sternum. Place the other hand on the lower rib cage. Have the child inhale and note the outward movement of the upper abdominal wall and the lower rib cage. Have the child hold this position briefly and then exhale, noting the inward movements of the upper abdominal wall and lower rib cage. Have the child repeat this several times while he is standing, walking, sitting, or lying down.[9] Then instruct the child to do as follows:

1) Inhale slowly. Hold. Exhale slowly.
2) Inhale slowly. Hold. Exhale quickly.
3) Inhale quickly. Hold. Exhale slowly.
4) Inhale quickly. Hold. Exhale quickly.
5) Inhale quickly. Exhale quickly.
6) Pant (for a short time only).
7) Practice all exercises until habitual.
8) Phonate the vowel ä (arm) for four, six, eight, and ten seconds.
9) Practice step 8 until the student can sustain the vowel for twenty seconds.
10) Phonate other vowels in the same manner.
11) Phonate the voiced fricatives in the same manner.
12) Produce the voiceless fricatives in the above manner.
13) Practice going from a whisper to a voice position on the vowel ä (arm).
14) Practice going from a whisper to a voice on all vowels.
15) Practice going from a voiceless to a voiced position using the above sound.
16) Practice an easy starting and stopping of the vowel tract with the sound 'a': Example – ä – ä – ä.
17) Use other vowels as in the exercise above.
18) Practice using varying degrees of loudness with steps 12, 16, and 17 above.

19) Practice the exercises while the child is walking, standing, sitting, and lying down.
20) Have the child pretend that he is the North Wind. Have him start with a whisper and gradually increase the sound 'oo' (moon) as the wind becomes stronger.
21) Practice saying one, two, and three words with one breath. Increase to ten words. Be certain to use words from the child's vocabulary that do not contain stuttering patterns.
22) Draw on the chalkboard five closed boxes, varying the size from small to large. Instruct the child to use the words "open me" in a voice which corresponds to the size of the box.
23) Draw a series of balloons and place numbers from one through twelve inside—increase the size of the numbers. Have the child make his voice louder as he counts. (Example: 1 2 3 4 5 6 7 8 9 10 11 12).
24) Place the following numbers on the board and instruct the child to produce a voice which corresponds to the size of the numbers.

    a. 1 2 3 4 5 6 7 8 9 10
    b. 1 2 3 4 5 6 7 8 9 10
    c. 1 2 3 4 5 6 7 8 9 10
    d. 1 2 3 4 5 6 7 8 9 10
    e. 1 2 3 4 5 6 7 8 9 10

25) Practice saying phrases and sentences of varying length. Again, these should be carefully selected to avoid any patterns that might cause stuttering. Arrange the carrier phrases as follows:

    □ □ The weather
    □ □ □ □ is warm
    □ □ □ □ □ □ in Detroit
    □ □ □ □ □ □ □ □ □ especially during July.

26) Practice lightly saying sentences with variations of loudness to convey different meanings.
27) Practice saying sentences with variations of stress and rhythm.
28) Practice blowing exercises that involve long, rhythmical movements.
29) Avoid any form of spasmodic exhalation in all the practices. Spasmodic breathing produces poor phrasing and rhythm of movement.

In response to these exercises the respiratory mechanism is shifted from conscious to automatic activation to regulate the depth and frequency of breathing in all situations of oral communication.

Phonation

Phonation takes place in the larynx and determines the pitch of the vocal tone produced. In working with the stutterer the therapist should attempt to extend the child's pitch range, increase the variation in pitch within that range, and train him to start and stop the vibration on different pitch levels, using varying degrees of force.[10]

An important part of this section is auditory training. Under ordinary listening conditions, the human organism is called upon to recognize, distinguish between, and interpret sounds that fall into three main categories: gross sounds, musical sounds, and speech sounds. Gross sounds encompass all the sounds common to the home, neighborhood, nature, and animals. Musical sounds are prevalent in the environment through the television, radio, and religious rituals. The most important aspect of musical sound is rhythm, which is as important in speech as it is in music. In the speech sounds category there are roughly sixteen vowels and twenty-five consonants that have basic symbolic value. It is imperative that the student be familiar with the basic sound patterns as described above, because good voice and speech are dependent upon them. Also, it will be easier to develop and maintain the desired goals if the child has an awareness of these categories.

The following procedures are designed to improve flexibility and rhythm patterns. The student should practice these procedures until he has overcome any difficulty in producing the desired melody (variations in pitch) and rhythm (variations in stress).

1) Have the child distinguish between high, middle, and low tones. (These tones can be produced by a toy xylophone, piano, or by the therapist.)
2) Use a xylophone or music maker and have the student reproduce the sound.
3) Play or reproduce sounds of the local environment and have the student identify the pitch of the sounds heard.
4) Say the ä (arm) sound softly. Have the child open his mouth wide and not move the tongue during phonation.
5) Say the ä (arm) sound while going from a low to a high pitch. Example:

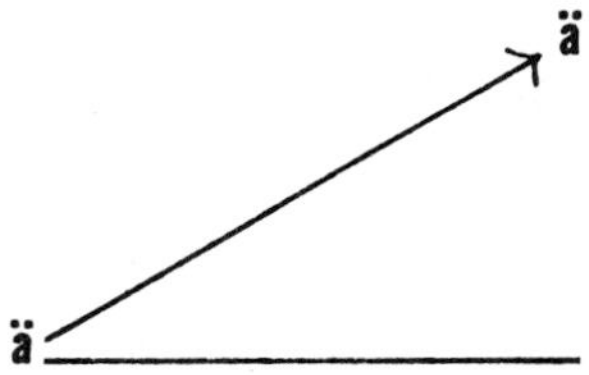

6) Use the same vowel and go from a high to a low pitch. Example:

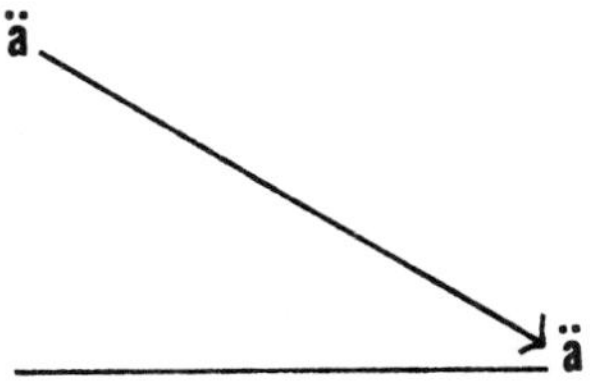

7) Use all long vowels in the same manner.
8) Raise and lower the pitch on one breath. Example:

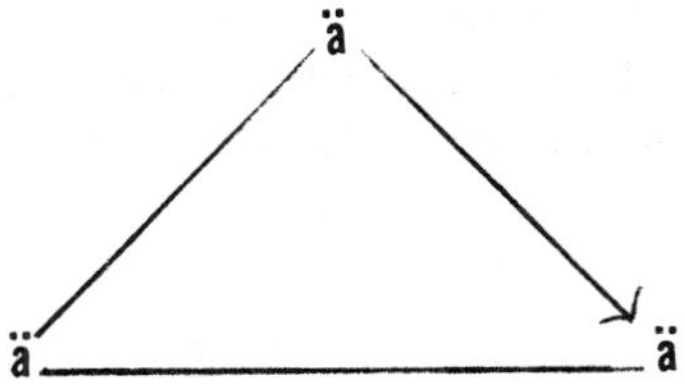

9) Have the child do the above practice with other vowels. Example:

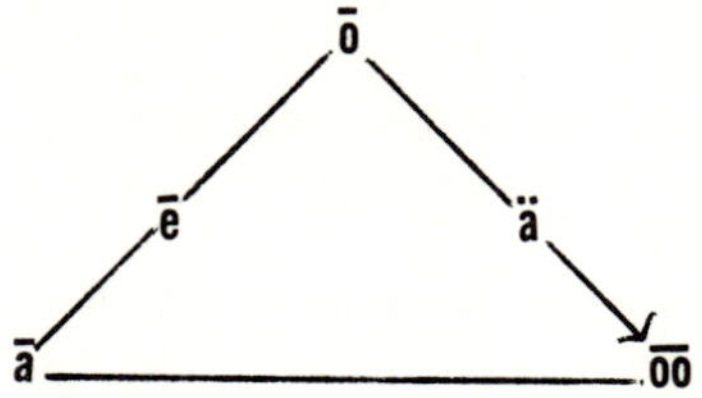

10) Have the child practice voice steps with vowels while going from a low to a high pitch and a high pitch to a low one. Example:

	(1)	(2)	(3)	(4)
High	ä	ä	ä	ä
			ä	ä
		ä		ä
Middle	ä	ä	ä	ä
		ä		ä
				ä
			ä	ä
Low	ä	ä	ä	ä

11) Practice the above, using other vowels.
12) Practice step 8, using voiced consonants.
13) Draw ten balloons on the board, extending from a low to a high pitch. Write the numbers one to ten on the balloons. (Color the balloons if child is unable to identify numbers.) Example:

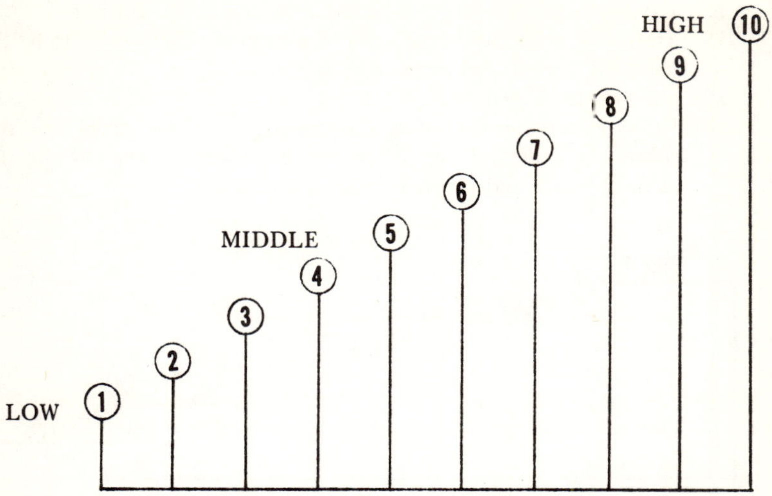

14) Reverse the order of the numbers.
15) Repeat step 11, but go from a high pitch to a low pitch.
16) Using the same format, arrange eight balloons for voice step practice to correspond with the following design.
Example:

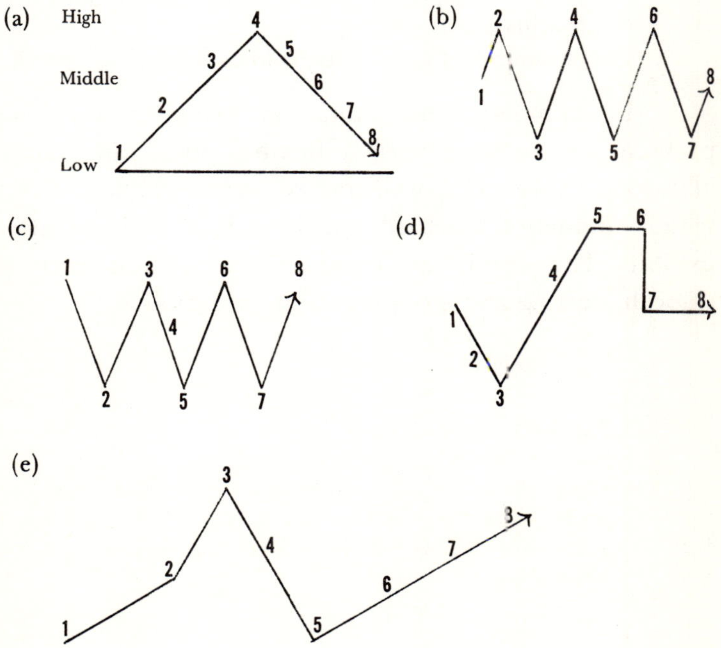

17) Use a voiced fricative consonant with the above format.
18) Start and stop the vocal cord vibration on different pitch levels using all vowels and consonant sounds.
19) Use words in step 18.
20) Draw a picture of some stair steps. Have the child say short sentences while putting the words on different steps of the stairs as he goes up and down in pitch patterns.

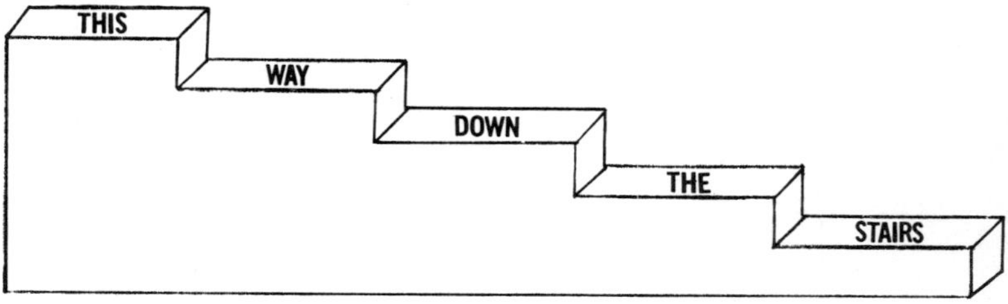

21) Vary the above exercises, using different degrees of loudness with the pitch change.
22) Practice saying phrases and sentences with a variation of inflections and stresses.
23) Practice saying sentences with emphasis on meaning.
24) Have the child tell a story and dramatize the characters by speaking in a high pitch for young persons and a deep voice for older persons.
25) Use controlled voice patterns in conversational speech.

In summary, the phonation exercises were designed to provide the stutterer with a flexible pitch range and a normal vibratory cycle. The well-trained voice exhibits a soft attack, which eliminates the hard attack on sounds that stutterers often exhibit. The child can compare this action with that of a smooth starting and stopping of an automobile.

Resonation

The coupling of the resonating cavities and the directing of the breath stream are major determinants of the voice quality. This unit deals with the procedure necessary to acquire normal voice qualities. For these practices it is important that the child use the conscious controls of the respiration and phonation units.

Basic to the acquisition of normal voice qualities is auditory training. Various qualities of sound can be demonstrated or played from recordings. These include rattles, clangs, thunder, growls, roars, echoes, tearing paper, shuffling feet, marching, and howling wind. The procedure involves playing or creating the selected sound for identification. Later the sounds are produced without identification, and the student is expected to make immediate recall of the sound.

The practices which follow have been found to be excellent in making the transition to correct voice patterns. This unit uses puppets, marionettes, comics, toys, and sound games as aids in the training program.

1) Have the child whisper short messages.
2) Produce the sounds of known animals.
3) Make the animals "speak" to one another.
4) Have the child imitate his favorite animal's voice, making the voice grow larger.

5) In a farmer's field there is a flock of sheep. A lamb has strayed from its mother. Direct the student to make the ba͝a sound loud enough for the mother sheep to hear her baby.
6) Have the child pretend that he is a policeman. There is an accident on a busy street, and he must get to the scene in a hurry. Have him produce a voice that would allow him to go through the traffic.
7) Ask the child to pretend that he is camping in the forest and wild animals are all around the tent. Have him produce a voice that will scare the animals away.
8) Direct the child to take the role of a member of his family and imitate the voice quality of the member selected.
9) Have the child play the part of a store manager for a pet or toy store when some children enter. How might the conversation go?
10) Have the student assume the role of club leader. How might he direct the activity? (Use the Brownies, Cub Scouts, or neighborhood clubs which are appropriate for the child's age.)
11) Practice reciting the stories of "Goldilocks and the Three Bears" and "The Three Little Pigs." Use a different voice for each character.
12) Put on a play or skit and assign roles to the students.
13) Use comics and have the student portray various characters.
14) Have the student describe or imitate other children's voices (the imitation of other class members is prohibited).
15) Play an instrumental music recording and have the child identify the various instruments.

In summary, this unit on resonation provides the child with structured exercises designed to develop the ability to use various voice qualities. Further, this unit should make the child's voice more responsive to thought and feeling through the skills acquired in the previous sections on respiration and phonation. Fundamentally, a person speaks by modulating the flow of air which passes from the lungs through the windpipe, vocal cords, throat, nose, and mouth cavities.

Articulation

At this phase the therapist should be concerned with the modification of the voiced and voiceless airstream to produce the various sounds of the language.

In preparing exercises for this section it at first seemed advisable to present the sounds as they occur in Visible Speech classifications. However, the Webster system has been substituted for the phonetic system of notation, because the child probably is more familiar with it. The sounds are listed and produced as follows:[11]

Group I—the voiceless stop sounds—p, t, and k; *Group II*—the voiced stop sounds—b, d, and g.

The p and b are produced by: stopping the breath stream by closing the nasal port and lips; building up voiceless or voiced breath pressure in the closed oral cavity; exploding the voiceless or voiced breath by quickly opening the lips.

The t and d are produced by: stopping the breath stream by placing the tip of the tongue against the gums (alveolar ridge) of the upper front teeth, while placing the sides of the tongue against the side teeth and closing the opening between the nose and throat; building up voiceless or voiced breath pressure in the closed oral cavity; exploding the voiceless or voiced breath by quickly moving the tongue tip away from the gums.

The k and g are produced by: stopping the breath stream

by placing the back of the tongue against the roof of the mouth and closing the opening between the throat and nose; building up voiceless or voiced breath pressure in the closed oral cavity; exploding the voiceless or voiced breath by quickly moving the tongue away from the roof of the mouth.

Group III—the voiceless fricatives—h, f, th^b, s, and sh; *Group IV*—the voiced fricative sounds—ɦ, v, th^v, z, and zh.

The h and ɦ are produced by: forming a small or restricted opening between the vocal cords at some point in the region of the glottis; closing the opening between the throat (pharyngeal) and the nasal cavities; emitting a continuous voiceless or voiced breath stream through the restricted opening.

The f and v are produced by: forming a small or restricted opening between the upper teeth and lower lip; closing the opening between the throat (pharyngeal) and the nasal cavities; emitting a continuous stream of voiceless or voiced breath through the restricted opening.

The th^b and th^v are produced by: forming a small or restricted opening between the tip of the tongue and the upper teeth; closing the opening between the throat (pharyngeal) and nasal cavities; emitting the voiceless or voiced breath stream through the restricted opening.

The s and z are produced by:[12] closing the nasal port; keeping the lips spread a little; keeping the teeth slightly apart; being sure that the sides of the tongue touch the sides of the upper teeth; grooving the tongue and placing the tongue tip against the ridge above the upper front teeth for the upper positions or behind the lower teeth for the lower positions; emitting the voiceless or voiced air stream through the grooved position of the tongue across the cutting edge of the teeth.

The sh and zh are produced by: forming a wide, shallow opening between the flattened tongue tip and the anterior palate; placing the sides of the tongue against the teeth and teeth ridge to direct the breath stream through the wide shallow opening; having a narrow opening between the upper and lower teeth; opening the lips and rounding them a little; closing the nasal port; emitting a continuous voiceless or voiced breath stream through the wide shallow groove against the cutting edge of the teeth and through the cavity formed by the lips.

Group V—the vowel and vowel-like sounds—ē, ǐ, ĕ, ă, *ȧ*, ä, ŏ, ȯ, ô, o͝o, o͞o, ẽr, ŭ, ȧ, y, w, l, r, m, n, ng.

These sounds are produced by the emission of the voiced breath through the different combinations of the coupled vocal cavities. The exact procedures for producing the vowels and vowel-like sounds of this group are as follows:

The ē sound (he) is produced by: closing the nasal port; opening the mouth just a little; spreading the lips slightly; touching the sides of the front of the tongue against the teeth; keeping the top of the tongue down flat; keeping the front of the tongue raised upward, leaving a narrow opening between the front of the tongue and the front of the roof of the mouth; using the voice without moving the lips, tongue, or jaw.

The ǐ sound (it) is produced by: closing the nasal port; opening the lips and jaw just a little more than for the ē with a reduction in the lip spread; touching the sides of the tongue against the sides of the upper teeth; placing the tip of the tongue down a little more than for the ē, and keeping it flat; leaving an opening between the front of the tongue and the front of the roof of the mouth; using the voice without moving the lips, tongue, or jaw.

The ĕ sound (met) is produced by: closing the nasal port; opening the lips and jaw just a little more than for the ǐ; placing the sides of the middle of the tongue against the sides of the upper teeth; spreading the tip of the tongue behind the lower front teeth and keeping it flat while leaving a slightly larger opening than for the ǐ; using the voice without moving the lips, tongue, or jaw.

The ă sound (at) is produced by: closing the nasal port; opening the lips and jaw a little more than for ĕ; placing the sides of the back of the tongue against the sides of the upper teeth; placing the tip of the tongue down while keeping it flat with a slightly larger opening than for the ē between the front of the tongue and the front of the roof of the mouth; using the voice without moving the lips, tongue, or jaw.

The ȧ sound (ask) is produced by: closing the nasal port; opening the lips and jaw a little more than for ă; flattening the tip of the tongue and elevating it slightly with the sides in contact with the lower front teeth; having the middle part of the tongue arched upward toward the hard palate; using the voice without moving lips, tongue, or jaw.

The ä sound (father) is produced by: closing the nasal port; opening the lips and jaw wide; keeping the tongue almost flat in the floor of the mouth; keeping the tip of the tongue down behind the lower front teeth; using the voice without moving lips, tongue, or jaw.

The ŏ sound (not) is produced by: closing the nasal port; opening the jaw wide; placing the lips in position for the ä, but rounded slightly; having the tongue position similar to the ä sound, except that the tongue is drawn farther backward and upward; producing the voice without using lips, tongue, or jaw.

The ō̇ (obey) sound is produced as a half-long ō by: closing the nasal port; opening the jaw for the ō position with rounded lips in a noticeable protrusion; keeping the tongue tip depressed while the back is further elevated and retracted toward the soft palate as in ô rising voice; not moving the lips, tongue, or jaw.

The ô sound (all) is produced by: closing the nasal port; opening the jaw wide; opening the lips wide bringing the corners forward toward the middle; placing the tip of the tongue behind the lower front teeth; keeping the tongue tip down and back a little in the floor of the mouth; keeping the back of the tongue up a little; using voice without moving the lips, tongue, or jaw.

The o͝o sound (book) is produced by: closing the nasal port; opening, rounding, and pushing the lips forward a little; opening the jaw a little less than for the ô; placing the tongue tip behind the lower front teeth; keeping the front of the tongue down and back; keeping the back of the tongue up and a little forward with the sides touching the upper teeth leaving a small opening; using voice without moving lips, tongue, or jaw.

The o͞o sound (moon) is produced by: closing the nasal port; rounding the lips and pushing them forward; placing the tongue tip down behind the lower front teeth; keeping the front of the tongue down and back; placing the back of the tongue up near the back of the roof of the mouth with the sides touching the upper teeth leaving a small opening; using voice without moving lips, tongue, or jaw.

The ŭ sound (up) is produced by: closing the nasal port; opening the jaw a little; placing the tongue tip behind the lower front teeth; keeping the tongue flat in mouth (the middle of the tongue may be raised just a little); using voice without moving the lips, tongue, or jaw.

The *ȧ* sound (sof*ȧ*) is produced by: closing the nasal port; opening the jaw and lips in a relaxed position; keeping the tongue on the floor of the mouth; using an unstressed voice without moving the lips, tongue, or jaw.

The ẽr sound (water) is produced by: closing the nasal port; keeping the lips and teeth slightly apart without rounding the lips; widening the tongue tip and curling it up and back without touching the roof of the mouth; placing the sides of the middle of the tongue against the sides of the upper teeth; using voice without moving the lips, tongue, or jaw.

The m sound (my) is produced by: opening the port between the nasal and throat cavities; maintaining a light closure at the lips; emitting a continuous stream of voiced breath through the nasal cavity.

The n sound (no) is produced by: opening the nasal port; maintaining a closure in the oral cavity as in the stop phase of d; emitting a continuous stream of voiced breath through the nasal cavity.

The ng sound (sing) is produced by: opening the port between the nasal and throat cavities; maintaining a closure by placing the back of the tongue against the posterior hard palate and part of the soft palate as in the stop phase of the g; emitting a continuous stream of voiced breath through the nasal cavity.

The w sound (we) is produced by: rounding the lips, without too much tension, to a position similar to that used in saying o͞o—(boot); raising the back of the tongue toward the palate to a position similar to that used in saying o͞o as in (boot); closing the nasal port; emitting a continuous stream of voiced breath while the articulators are moving toward their position for the combined adjacent sound.

The y sound (you) is produced by: placing the lips in approximately the same position as for ĭ—(it); starting with the other articulators held almost in the ē (eve) position, except that the elevated portion of the tongue is higher and not so far forward in the mouth; closing the opening between the throat and nasal cavities; emitting a continuous stream of voiced breath while the articulators are moving toward their positions for the combined adjacent sound.

The r (red) sound is produced by: starting with the mouth open as in making t with slight rounding of the lips; broadening the tongue tip and curling it up and back toward the center of the hard palate, but not touching or by moving the tip of the tongue forward from an elevated position near the center of the palate toward the alveolar ridge; closing the nasal port; emitting a continuous stream of voiced breath while the articulators are moving toward or away from the r position.

The l sound (look) is produced by: assuming the position of the lips similar to the lip position for ŭ—(up); placing the tip of the tongue in contact with the alveolar ridge or adjacent hard palate, depending upon the l being produced; holding the sides of the front of the tongue against the upper front teeth; maintaining openings between the back sides of the tongue and the upper molars on each side of the mouth; closing the nasal port; emitting a continuous stream of voiced breath while the articulators are moving toward the positions of the combined adjacent sounds.

The above description applies to the initial glide (l). When the tongue tip is in contact with the alveolar ridge, it is in the position for the front l. When the tongue is retracted and the tip is in contact with the anterior hard plalate, the position is that for the back l. In a broad sense, the front l position is used with the front vowels and the back (l) position is used with the back vowels. Too, in the glide (l), the moving of the articulators predominates, while in the production of the other l's the steady state phase may predominate.

Group VI—combinations of sounds ā, ī, ō, ū, oi, ou, hw, ch, j.

This group involves the production and combining of sounds within a group such as ä and i for l, or the combining of sounds from two groups, such as t and sh for the production of the ch sound. The latter is an example of Group I and III combinations.

The ā sound (say) is produced by: combining the ȧ and ĭ sounds; stopping the voice and movement of the tongue, lips, and jaw at the same time.

The i sound (eye) is produced by: combining the ä and ĭ sounds; starting in the a position and moving quickly to the i position; stopping the voice and the movement of the tongue, lips, and jaw at the same time.

The ō sound (go) is produced by: combining the ȯ and o͝o sounds; starting at the ȯ position and moving quickly to the o͝o position; stopping the voice and movement of the tongue, lips, and jaw at the same time.

The ū sound (use) is produced by: combining the ĭ and o͞o sounds; starting in ĭ position and moving quickly to the o͞o position; stopping the voice and movement of the tongue, lips, and jaw at the same time.

The oi sound (oil) is produced by: combining the ô and ĭ sounds; starting at the ô position and moving quickly to the ĭ position; stopping the voice and movement of the tongue, lips, and jaw at the same time.

The ou sound (out) is produced by: combining the ä and o͝o sounds; starting at the ä position and quickly moving to the o͝o position; stopping the voice and movement of the tongue, lips, and jaw at the same time.

The hw sound (where) is produced by: opening the jaw a little, with rounded and extended lips, similar to that for o͞o–(boot); placing the back of the tongue near the back of the roof of the mouth leaving a small opening; placing the tongue tip down and back of the front teeth; directing the breath out of the mouth through the small opening; producing a voiceless h preceding a partially unvoiced w–(we); moving the articulators to the vowel that follows as the w phase is blended with that vowel.

The ch sound (church) is produced by: combining the t and sh sounds; starting at the t position and quickly moving the tongue to the sh position while letting out the breath that was built up for the stop phase of t; continuing to let out the sound while moving to the next sound.

The j sound (judge) is produced by: combining the d and zh sounds; starting at the d position and quickly moving to the zh position while using voice; continuing to use voice while moving to the next sound.

This approach to the development of a correct system of teaching articulation represents the most concise and accurate physiological functions of the muscles of articulation, which include the lips, facial muscles, jaws, teeth, tongue, hard palate, soft palate, and the pharynx. In working with the stutterer the therapist's goal is to exercise the muscle groups used in articulation to increase their rate, range, strength, and accuracy of coordinated movement. This permits the establishment of new oral positions from which sounds can be produced without stuttering. Further, it is essential to combine the acquired skills of respiration, phonation, and resonation for success in the unit that follows. All movements must be accurate and well timed.

LIP EXERCISES:

The child should move the lips from a smiling to whistling

position or ē → o͞o; pull up one side of the lips, then the other; move the lips from positions of slightly closed to open; place lips into position for bilabial sounds; increase the above exercises from a slow to a rapid rate of movement; practice daily until normal habit patterns are established.

JAW EXERCISES:

The child should move the jaw from side to side; move the jaw forward and backward; move the jaw up and down in a chewing fashion, but be careful not to touch the teeth; move the jaw around and around; practice going from a slow to rapid rate of movement; combine lip and jaw action for the bilabial sounds; practice the controls daily until new, normal habit patterns are established.

TONGUE EXERCISES:

The child should move the tongue in and out of the mouth; move the tongue from side to side; raise and lower the tongue while trying to touch the nose and chin with the tongue tip; move the tongue in a circular movement inside the lips; extend the tongue and point tip; extend the tongue and alternate movements of pointing and broadening; groove the tongue in and out of the mouth; dot tip of tongue along the lip margins; retract tongue tip while keeping sides against teeth; move the tongue tip from the upper teeth to the beginning of soft palate; practice daily until normal patterns are established; go from a slow to rapid rate of movement; practice moving the tongue through all sounds involving the tongue positions.

In the articulation exercises that are listed above, the

therapist can tell the child that his tongue can be a horse, a car, or an airplane. His lips can be the doors and his mouth can be the barn, garage, or hangar.

The vowels are presented at this juncture because they represent the basic movement of a syllable unit; and they have the least physiological resistance in production. The vowels listed in this manual carry the Webster symbols, since this method of orthography is used in most schools and the child is more likely to be familiar with it. He should practice these vowels until normal patterns are established.

FRONT VOWELS:

ē - me
ĭ - it
ĕ - bed
ă - at
ā - ask

BACK VOWELS:

ȧ - sof*a*
ä - are
ô - all
o͝o - foot
o͞o - moon

MID VOWELS:

ŭ - up
û - word
ẽr - mother

COMBINATION VOWELS (Diphthongs):

ā - May
ī - eye
ō - toe
ū - you
oi - oil
ou - out

The stutterer should practice these vowels in combination with other vowels, starting first with the combination of front and back vowels. Later he should use various combinations. The following list is suggestive of the procedure.

1. ē - ä ē - ä ē - ä - ā	2. ĭ - ô ĭ - ô ĭ - ô - ẽr	3. ĕ - o͝o ĕ - o͝o ĕ - o͝o - oi
4. ă - o͞o ă - o͞o ă - o͞o - ī	4. ē - o͞o ē - o͞o ē - o͞o - ou	6. ä - ā ä - ā ä - ā - ī
7. ī - o͞o ī - o͞o ī - o͞o - u	8. ĭ - ĕ ĭ - ĕ - o͞o	9. oi - ou oi - ou oi - ou - ă
10. ŭ - ä ŭ - ä ŭ - ä - ô	11. ā - oi ā - oi ā - oi - ô	12. o͞o - ẽr o͞o - ẽr o͞o - ẽr - ŭ
13. ō - ī ō - ī ō - ī - o͞o	14. o͞o - o͝o o͞o - o͝o o͞o - o͝o - ă	15. ẽr - ĕ ẽr - ĕ ẽr - ĕ - ă

For consonant practices the therapist should introduce all consonant sounds as found in the modulation groups presented in the beginning of this unit. To do this, he should: combine consonants for practice from different groups, example: (b - t), (p - v), (f - z); combine each sound with a schwa vowel, example: (bȧ - tȧ); (*a* as in sof*a)*; combine consonants in the same modulation group, example: (t - d), (s - z), (f - l - g), (m - v - z); combine each sound with a schwa vowel.

The nonsense syllable technique was invented by Ebbinghaus in 1885. A nonsense syllable consists of a vowel between two consonants, a meaningless unit of speech that does not form a word. It is used in this therapy to increase the functional efficiency of the speech musculature and to aid in auditory discrimination.

In 1928[13] Glaze calibrated nonsense syllables according to their association values—the ease with which they suggest words. These Glaze syllables are used here.

Bip	Dak	Nah	Koj	Mep
Yad	Kac	Quz	Des	Wog
Cug	Jof	Puh	Rij	Jaf
Bek	Heb	Dac	Yid	Pex
Cey	Xip	Zod	Mos	Mun
Fef	Tiz	Uab	Zar	Wob
Gak	Cay	Faw	Lav	Vav
Cag	Bif	Jos	Del	Vax
Vew	Pel	Les	Hun	Coz
Gan	Sol	Mel	Loy	Dub

The therapist should construct meaningful syllables by combining all the consonant sounds found in the practice above. To do this he should: combine the consonants with front vowels (Example: Pē, Pī, Pĕ, Pă); combine the consonants with the back vowels (Example: Pä, Pô, Po͝o, Po͞o); combine the consonants with the mid vowels (Example: Pŭ, Pe͠r); combine the consonants with the combination vowels (Example: Pā, Pī, Pō, Pū, Poi, Pou); combine consonant—vowel—consonant in steps 1, 2, 3, and 4 above; combine two or more syllables for syllable drills (Example: pŭ tŭ kŭ; bŭ, dŭ, gŭ; or pŭ, tŭ, kŭ, sŭ, thŭ); practice the above exercises with a variation in speed of utterance; repeat the exercises with a variation in loudness.

Consonant blends included in this unit represent a transitional movement from one consonant to another to release or terminate a meaningful articulation.[14] The releasing blends are:

Bl	Br	Dr	Dw	Fl	Gl
Gr	Kl	Kr	Kw	Pl	Pr
Shr	Sk	Skl	Skr	Skw	Sl
Sm	Sn	Sp	Spl	Spr	St
Str	Sw	Thr	Thw	Tr	Tw

Instruct the student to produce the above blends with all vowel patterns (Example: Bl = Blā, Blĕ, Bl$\overline{\text{oo}}$).

The terminating blends are:

Bd - rubbed	Lt - malt
Bz - dubs	Lv - twelve
Cht - pitched	Rb - disturb
Dz - adds	Rd - hard
Fs - puffs	Rf - scarf
Fth - fifth	Rj - large
Gd - rigged	Rk - lark
Gz - eggs	Rm - alarm
Jd - edged	Rp - carp
Nt - sent	Rs - scarce
Nth - tenth	Rsh - marsh
Nz - buns	Rt - port
Ngd - banged	Rth - mirth
Nk - sink	Rv - starve
Ps - tops	Rz - stars
Pt - apt	Sht - hushed
Ks - box	Sk - ask
Kt - act	Md - hummed
Lb - bulb	Mp - limp
Ld - schooled	Mt - exempt
Ldz - molds	Nz - bans
Lf - self	Nch - bunch
Lj - bulge	Nj - lunge
Lm - elm	Ns - ounce
Lp - help	Sp - asp
Ls - else	St - post
Lsh - welsh	Thd - bathed

Ts - lots		Zn - chosen	
Vz - loves		Zmz - myospasms	
Zd - raised			

Instruct the student to combine *all* vowel patterns with the terminal compound consonants (Example: Bd = ŭbd, ăbd, äbd).

Being aware of established controls, the student should practice saying the following numbers as directed.

1)	2)	3)	4)
1	3	2-5	1-3-4
2	1	3-6	3-2-5
3	2	8-1	6-8-1
4	4	8-7	5-9-8
5	6	6-3	2-4-2
6	5	4-9	7-1-3
7	8	5-8	4-7-6
8	9	1-6	9-8-9
9	10	2-3	5-5-3
10	7	7-2	5-7-2

5)	6)	7)
3-2-3-2	1-5-7-3-8	632-157
4-1-6-3	9-6-8-2-4	987-612
5-2-6-4	3-7-9-1-3	356-789
6-3-7-5	8-6-1-4-7	713-254
7-4-8-6	3-5-2-5-1	432-159
8-5-9-7	7-9-3-6-8	891-732
9-6-1-8	5-8-4-7-2	632-459
1-7-2-9	6-1-5-8-3	491-874
2-8-3-1	4-8-6-9-1	521-346
4-9-4-2	1-3-7-2-5	136-891

8) Instruct the student to vary the stress in the above exercises.
9) Instruct the student to vary the rate in the exercises.
10) Instruct the student to vary the force in the exercises.

The following exercises are advanced practiced forms of modulation groups. These sounds are produced without stopping the breath or voiced air stream, i.e., there is to be no hold on the sounds. Each sound when produced is flowed (blended into the one which follows).

f, th^{b}, s
v, th, z
sh, ch, zh
b, d, t,
g, k, j
w, l, r, z
t, w, l, n
h, s, f, p
p, d, s, b
z, h, f, l
b, v, q, n
v, l, d, sh
v, z, v, z
r, p, d, g
b, v, d, z

z, h, s, j, m, f
r, d, q, t, f, s
t, v, r, s, z, l
f, t, g, m, n, g
s, h, r, b, z, t
x, v, q, r, m, z
h, f, s, j, s, l
n, r, c, ch, zh, sh
p, l, t, v, n, d
b, w, f, z, m, f
d, v, z, l, v, z
th^{b}, z, th^{v}, m, b, g, n
m, t, h, s, k, b
l, p, y, th^{v}, d, g
h, s, r, z, y, j, ch

Make a longer list of consonants as in the example which follows: v, z, l, r, j, zh, d, m, n, th, f, s, t, b.
Combine consonants and numbers. Example: p, e, 5, v, z, b, 9, j, l, l, f, 7, z.
Combine consonants, numbers and vowels. Example: v, o, 5, z, 6, j, l, a, e, 7, i.
Change pitch on the voiced sounds in exercises 3, 4, 5, 6, and 7.
Change volume on the voiced sounds in the above groups.
Combine rate, pitch, and volume variations in the above groups.

Each of the following sentences contains a word with a sound missing. Instruct the child to supply the missing sound to complete the word. The purpose of this practice is auditory discrimination and vocabulary building. The child should maintain the controls learned in the previous units.

1) What letter placed before *ame* makes the name of something you can play? (g, t, l)
2) Place a letter before *ake* and you will have a garden tool. (r, w, k)
3) A letter before *ight* tells when the stars come out. (n, m, s)
4) What letter do you need before *ine* to tell you where copper comes from? (m, n, i)
5) What letter placed after *do* makes the name of an animal that barks? (g, k, b)
6) Put a letter before *air* and the new word tells what the barber cuts. (h, f, g)
7) What letter put before *rain* means a way to travel? (t, d, v)

8) What is the missing letter before *ate* which tells you what you open to get into your yard? (g, k, r)
9) What letter do you put after *was* to tell you what you do before eating? (h, th, f)
10) What does your father do when the lawn grass grows long? The word starts with m.
11) Put a letter to *ight* and *eat* to tell what we get from the sun. (l, h)
12) When the windows in your bedroom are not closed, they are what? (open)
13) In the story of "The Three Bears," what did they put their porridge in? (bowls)
14) Make the name of a cat's coat by supplying the missing letter in f - r. (u)
15) What does your mother do with her broom? (sweep)
16) Change *ice* to food by adding what sound? (r)
17) Name a color that is the same as a fruit. (grape, orange, peach)
18) Put a letter before *eer* and you will have my favorite animal. (d)
19) Change the word *arm* by adding a letter which tells where a farmer lives. (f)
20) What is the word that tells where teachers work? (school)
21) Change the flower *aster* to a holiday by putting a letter before it. (E)
22) What bird crows in the morning? (rooster, cock)
23) How is water carried into your house? (pipes)
24) What sound is missing in *uzz* that tells what sound a bee makes? (b)
25) What letter is missing in *oll* that tells what girls like to play with? (d)
26) Name the word that tells what we use on a rainy day to put over our heads? (umbrella)
27) What letter added to *oa* tells what a farmer feeds his horse? (t)
28) With what do we hear? (ears)
29) What is another name for our sight? (eyes)
30) What letter added to *boot* means more than one? (s)
31) Put three letters before *key* and you will have the bird of choice for Thanksgiving. (tur)
32) What word names something that puts out a fire? (water)
33) What is missing in *corn* that makes the name of a squirrel's delight? (a)
34) Put a letter after *clow* and you have a circus actor. (n)
35) Add a letter to *late* and it tells what we eat on. (p)
36) When I tell you something, you listen. If you wish to say something, I listen while you _ alk. (t) What is the letter? What is its sound?

In the following word discrimination game the child should say the word or words that will complete each sentence accurately. The purpose of this practice is auditory training. Here the student must recognize and identify the words with similar auditory characteristics.

1) We can hear a ______________.
bog - dog

2) Smokey is a ______________.
bear - pear

3) Nan went to the school ______________.
house - louse

4) Did you take the ______________ from the lock.
tea - key

5) ______________ out the door.
Book - Look

6) John came to a ______________.
top - stop - pot

7) He said, "We shall ______________ for ______________.
ran - run fun - sun

8) A frog ______________ on a ______________.
fell - tell log - hog

9) I ______________ time by the ______________ every ______________.
fell - tell lock - clock morning - norming

10) A bird was ______________ through the ______________ as I looked ______________ the ______________.
flying - tying - buying air - hair - stair out - in - into wind - window

Rhyming words provide for rhythmic movements of the articulators using one and two syllable words and will display the likeness between vowel elements in words. If the child is able to read, the therapist can write the words on the chalkboard as well as present them through oral discourse.

The single syllable words may be made up as follows:
at - bat - cat - fat - gat - hat - mat - pat - rat - sat - vat.
an - ban - can - jan - man - pan - ran - tan - van.
add - bad - cad - dad - fad - had - mad - sad.
Make other single-syllable rhyming words.

The two syllable words may be made up as follows:
bumped - lumped - humped - jumped.
castle - bustle - hustle - whistle.
delight - tonight - moonlight - sunlight.

The therapist should make other two syllable rhyming words and ask the student to vary the stress and rate of utterance in the above words.

Nursery rhyme practice is a continuation and more advanced exercise of the above unit. This practice treats speech as a complete rhythmical movement and prepares the approach to sentences and conversational speech patterns that will aid in making the new habits automatic. In this practice, the child, being aware of controls, should use gross muscle movements to accompany and set rhythms by clapping the hands or by using some other acceptable manner. For success in this unit, the child should learn the following nursery rhymes: Peas Porridge Hot; Jack Be Nimble; "Bow, Wow," Says the Dog; Pussycat, Pussycat; Little Jack Horner; Jack Sprat; Little Boy Blue; Jack and Jill; Rub - A - Dub - Dub; Ding, Dong Bell; Baa, Baa, Black Sheep; Ole King Cole; Humpty Dumpty; Old Mother Hubbard; Mary Had a Little Lamb.

WORDS, PHRASES, and SENTENCES:

There are approximately 5,000 words in the list in the Appendix of this volume (beginning p. 74). Most children when they enter school know at least 5,000 words, and some know many more. Therefore, the list is considered to be complete to meet any particular pattern likely to be encountered by the child in his first three years of school. The words are compiled from the Horn Kindergarten Word List, the 100-most-frequently-used-words lists, the Dolch and the Barnhart and Bloomfield[15] word lists. It is not the purpose of this unit to use all the words listed for any one student. However, they are provided here to aid the therapist in selecting words for oral practice which meet the needs of the child involved. The following is a general suggestion: assign a word and have the child produce it, using good articulation patterns; have the student put the word into a phrase (Example: using the word "active," an active boy); have the student put the word into a sentence (Example: He is an active boy); produce words, phrases, and sentences with varying degrees of loudness; using selected words, phrases, and sentences, vary the quality, inflection, stress, and rate to give different meanings to the utterances.

SPELLING AND READING:

This unit is included at this juncture in therapy to provide for cognitive-motor synthesis with written symbols. Combine all unit controls. Use both visual and dictative methods with words from the vocabulary list.

1) Begin spelling with a very slow rate and gradually increase the rate of utterance to the point of difficulty. Continue this type of practice until the student's rate has been extended below and beyond the normal pattern.
2) Change pitch with the above exercise.
3) Change volume with the spelling exercise.
4) Change rate, pitch, and volume in the above exercise. (Note: In step 1, slow the rate of utterance to the point where the student is able to produce sounds and movement without a visual or auditory evidence of a struggle with the letters involved.)
5) Read aloud, blending all words at a very slow rate.

6) Read aloud, going from a slow to rapid rate of utterance.
7) Read aloud on different pitch levels.
8) Read aloud on different volume levels.
9) Read aloud with rate, pitch, and volume shifts.
10) Practice reading and spelling exercises going from silent oral movements (Example: whisper to voice, and a variation of this practice whisper, voice, whisper, silent movements, whisper, voice, movements).

STORYTELLING:

This method of instruction employs conversational speech patterns. The child should make up and tell a story about each of the pictures on the following pages. The child is free to make up any story he wishes. The purpose of this practice is the development of structured speech patterns, which allow the child to apply controlled speech patterns from objective to subjective knowledge.

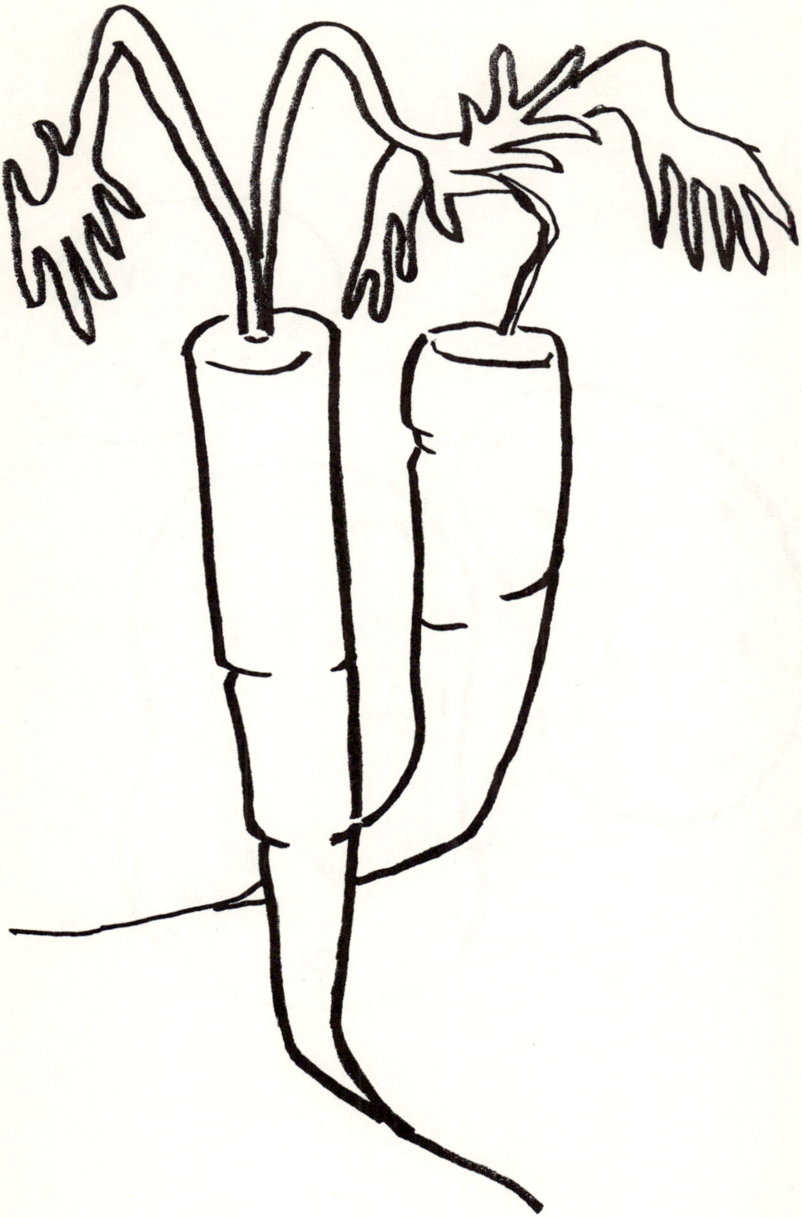

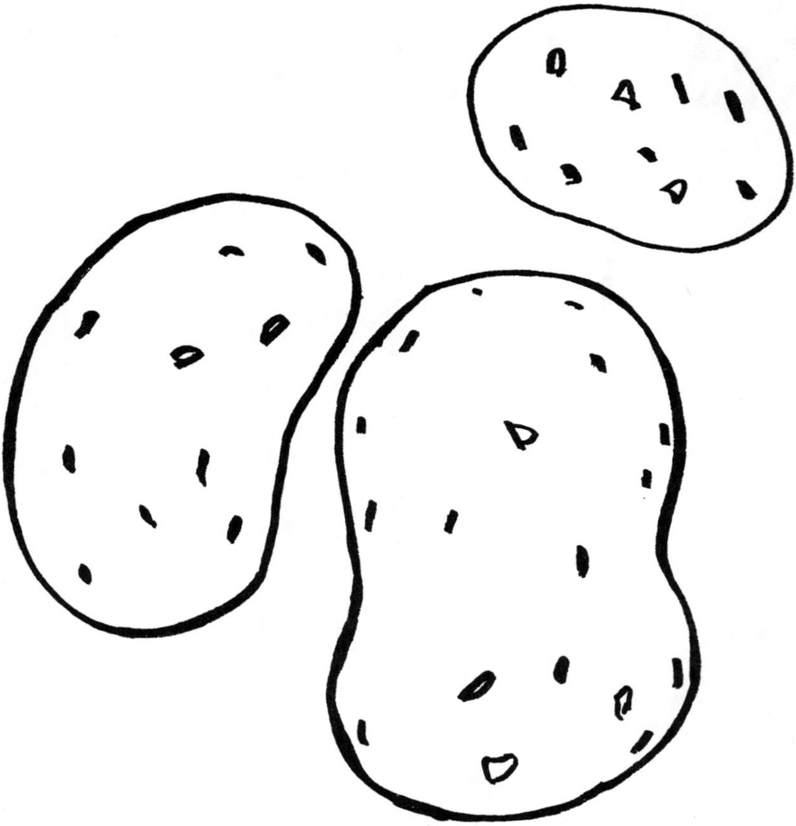

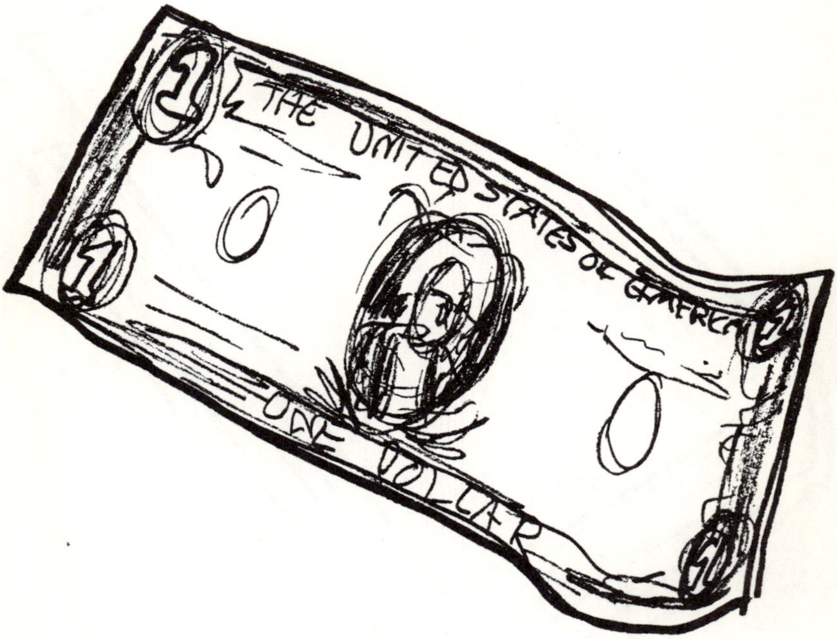
THE UNITED STATES OF AMERICA
ONE DOLLAR

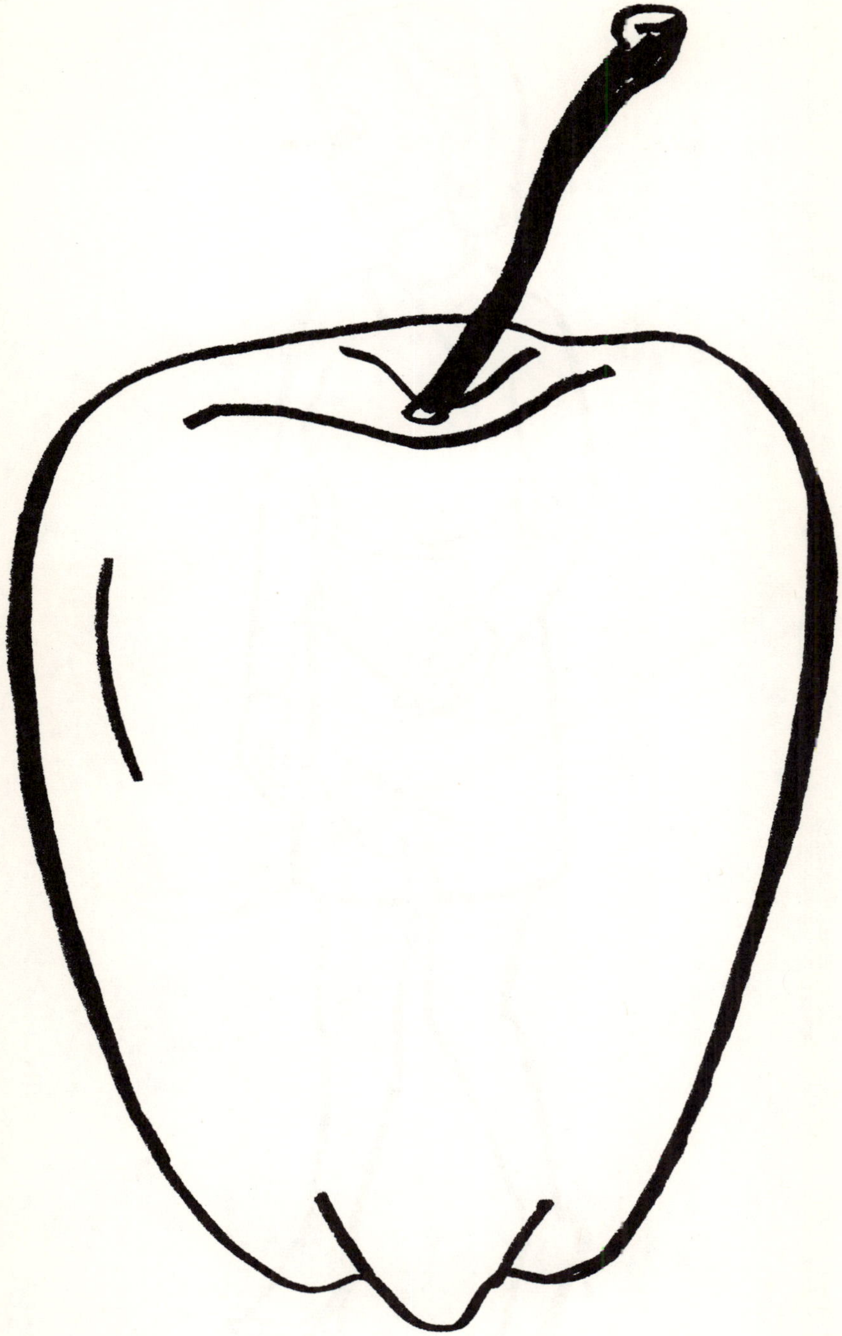

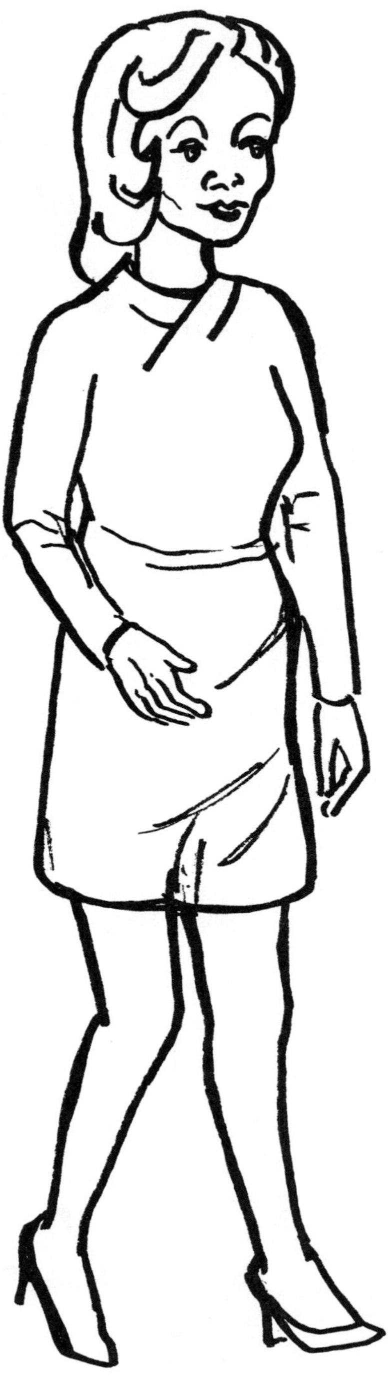

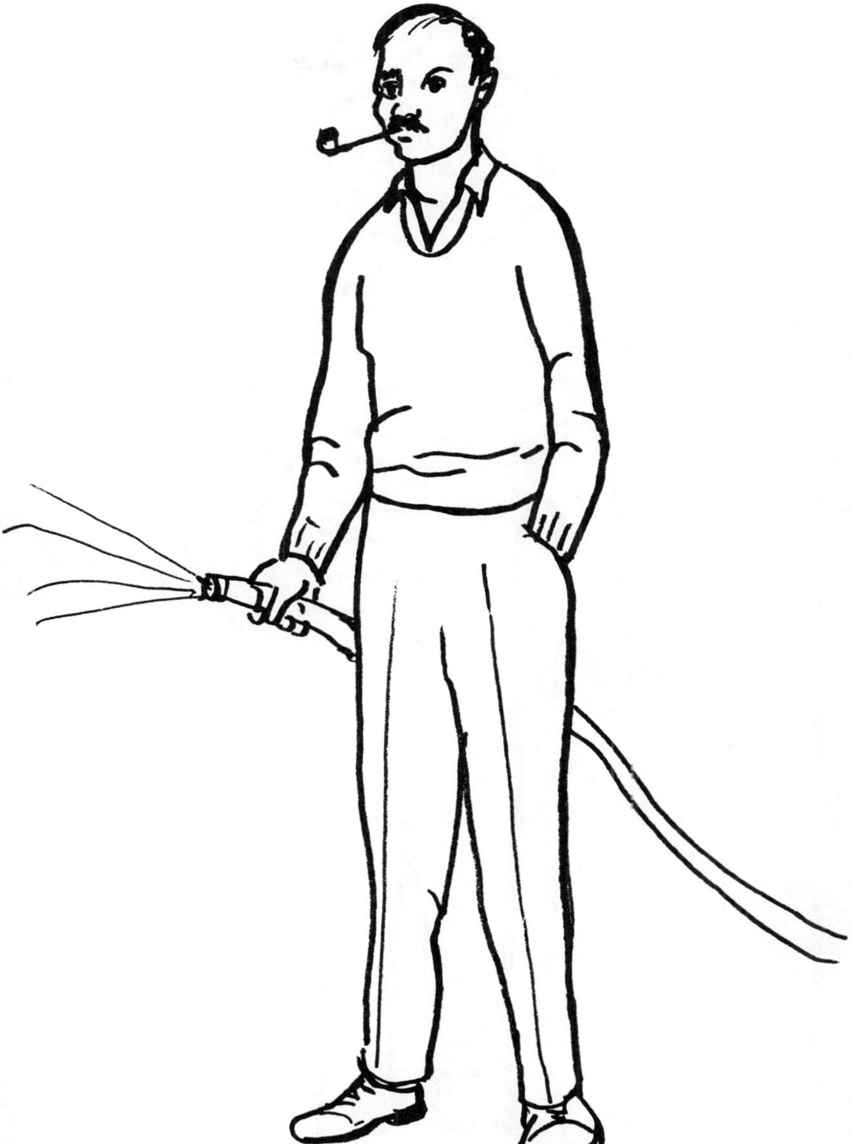

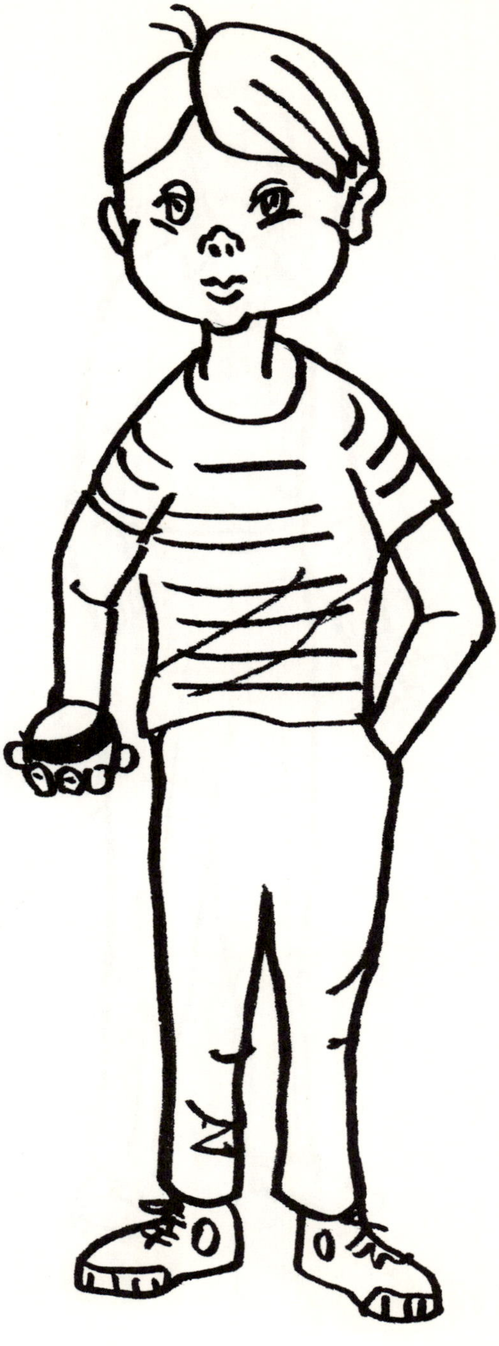

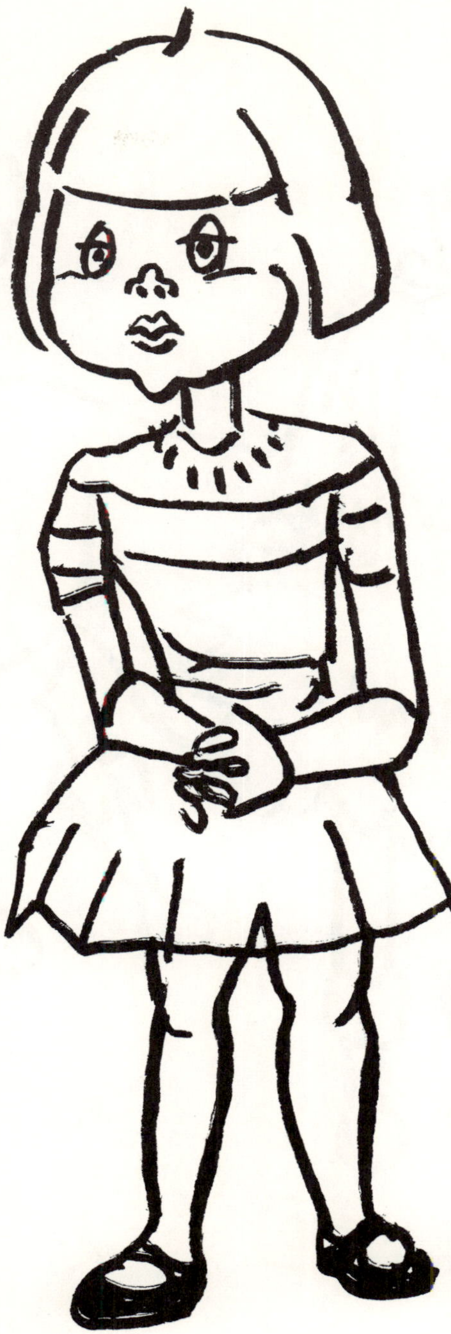

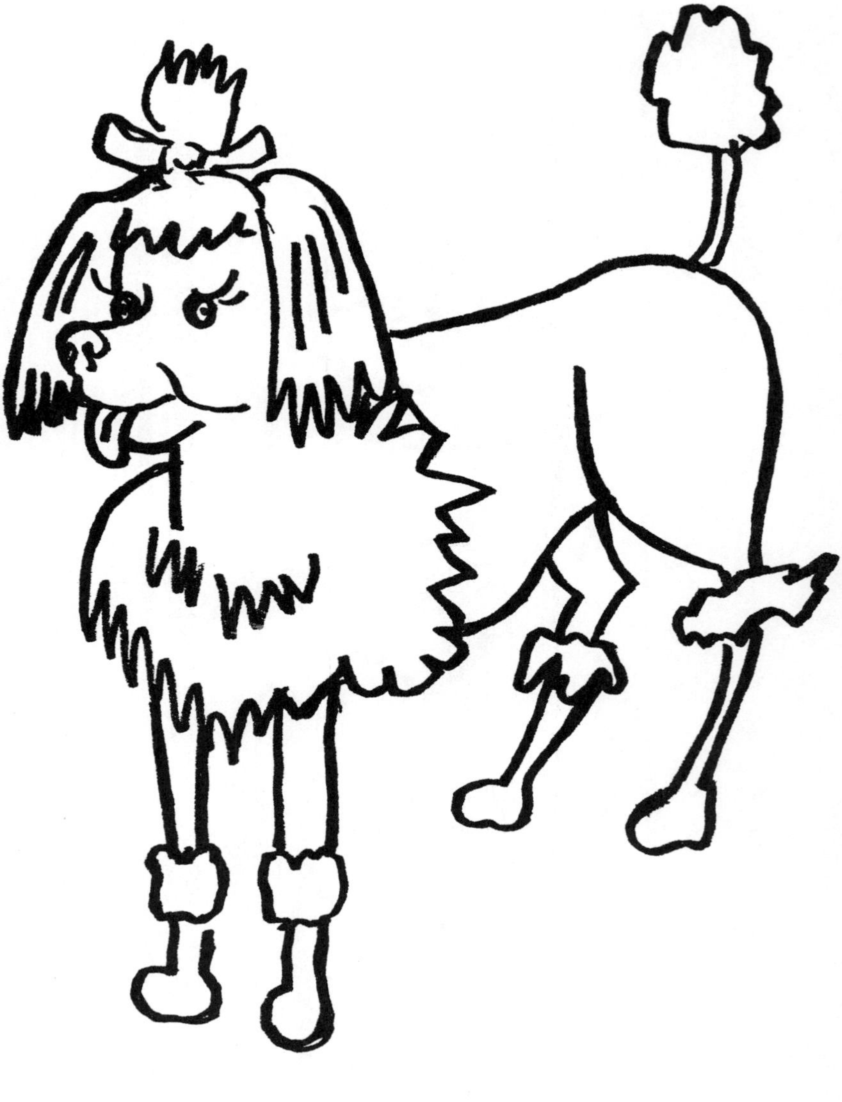

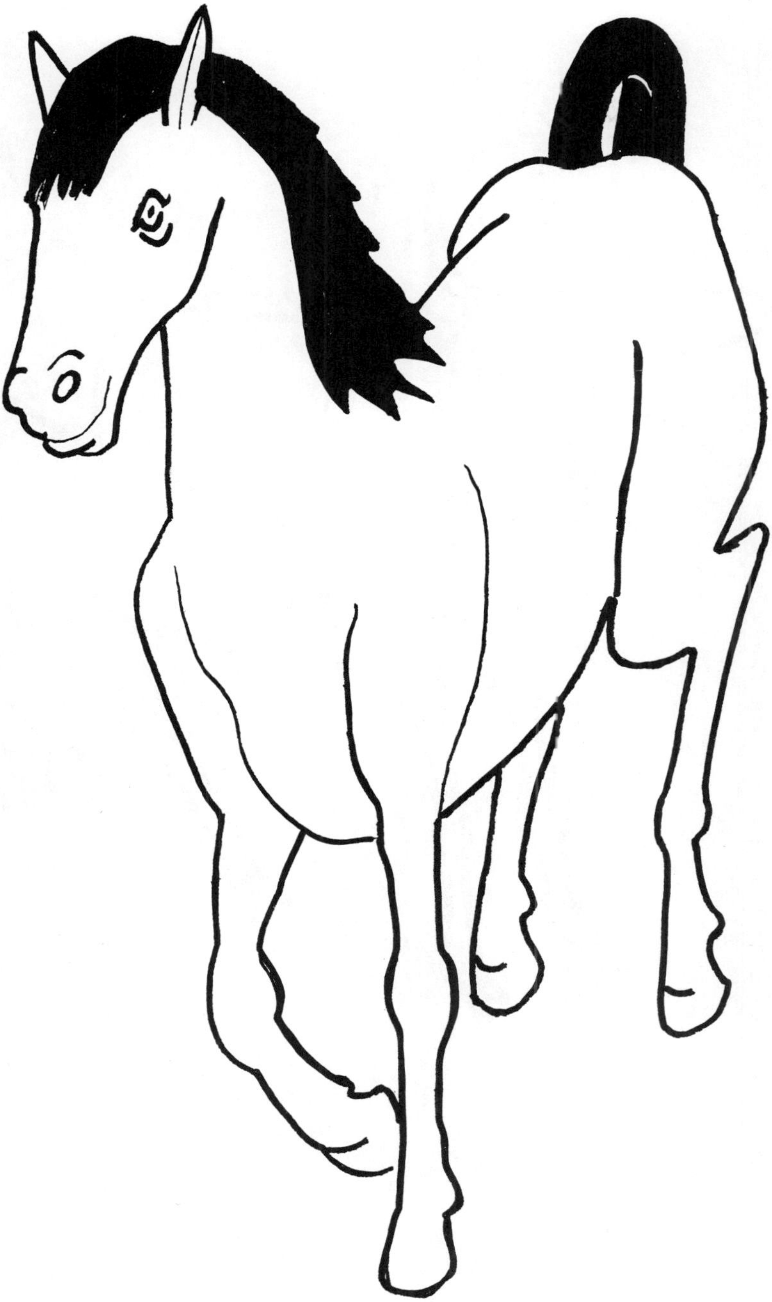

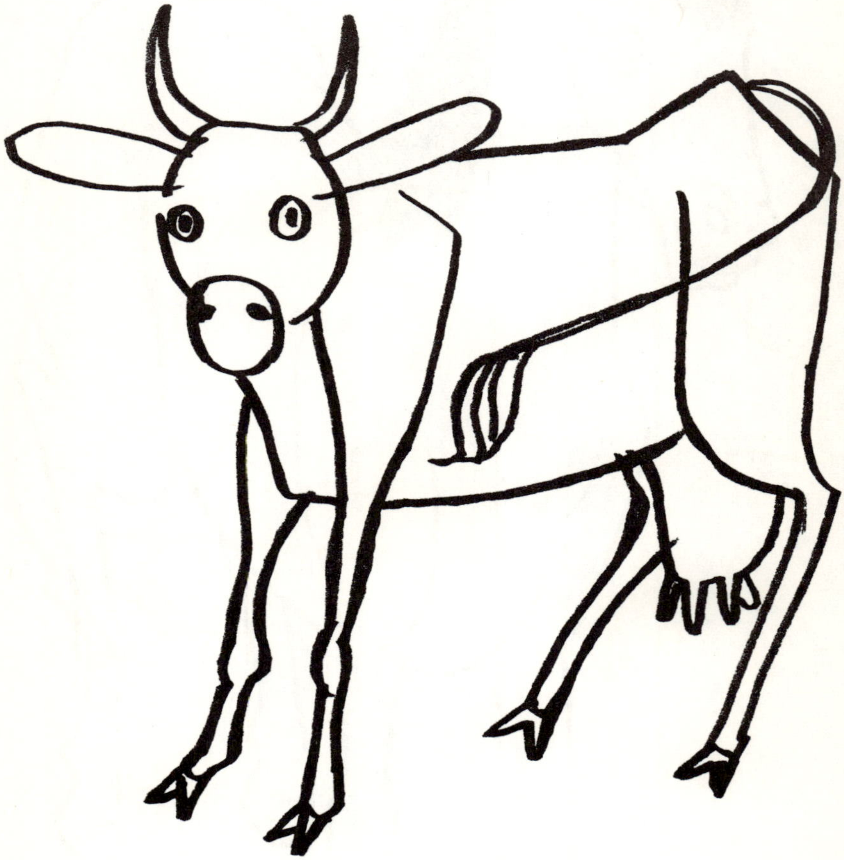

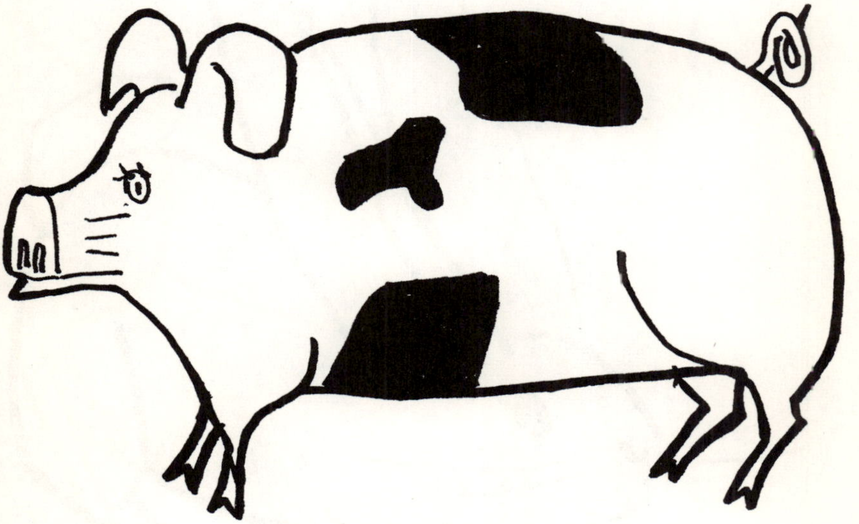

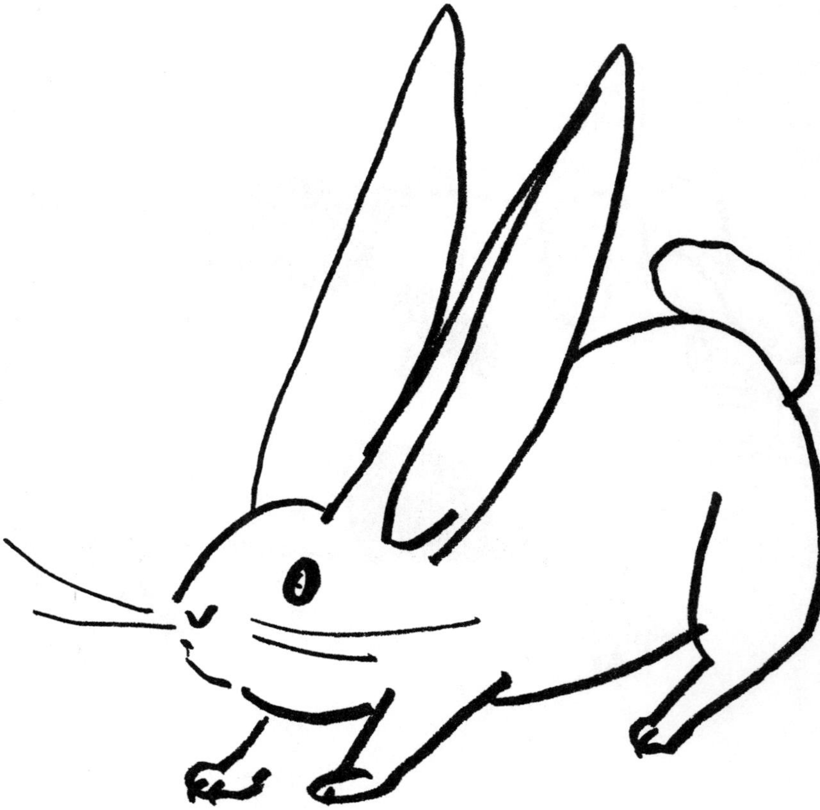

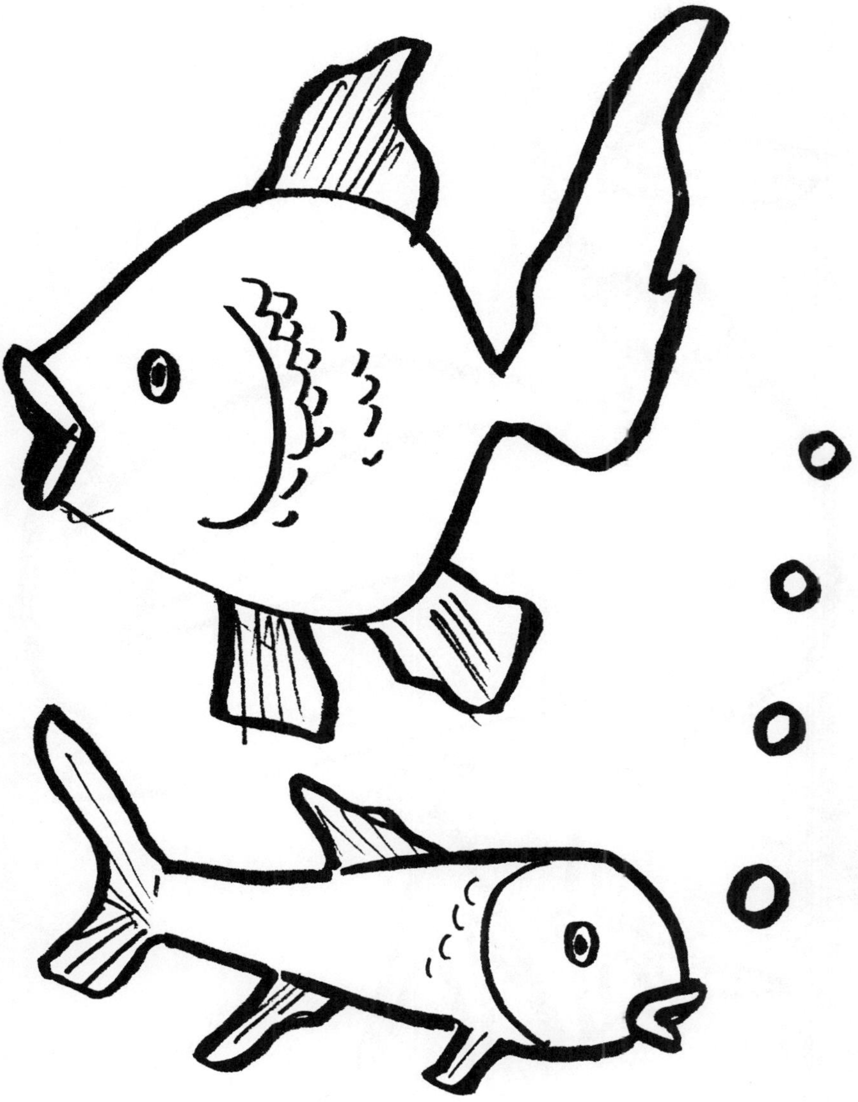

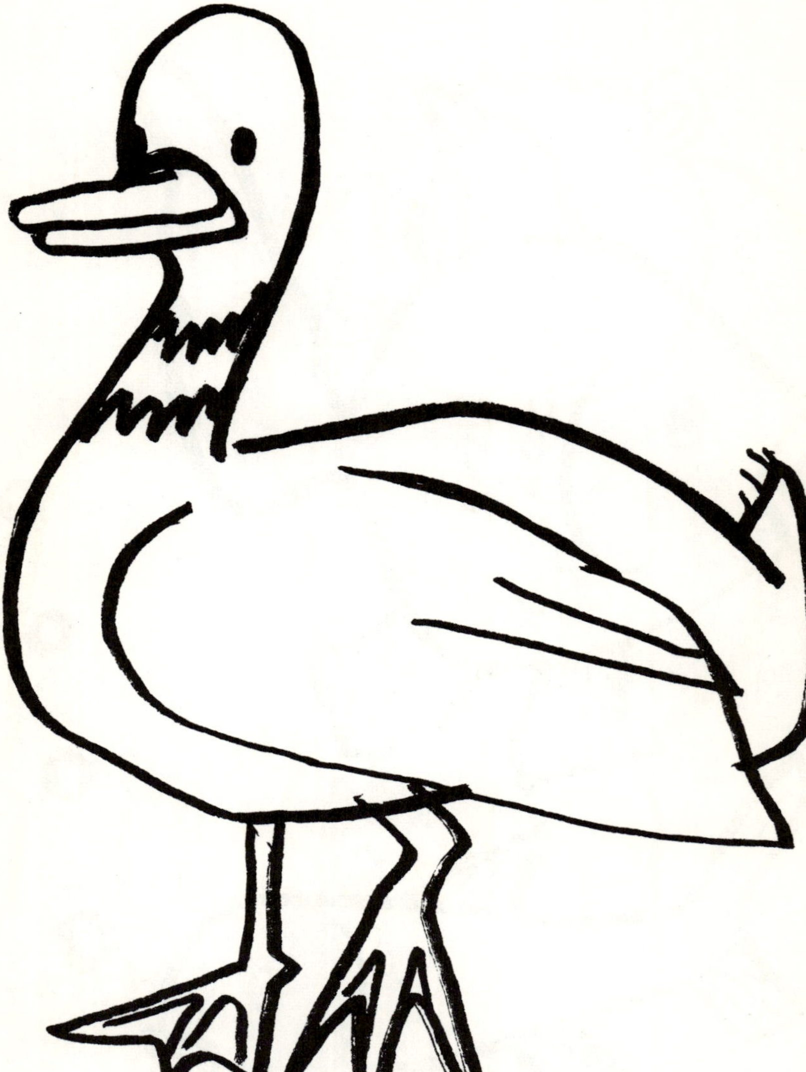

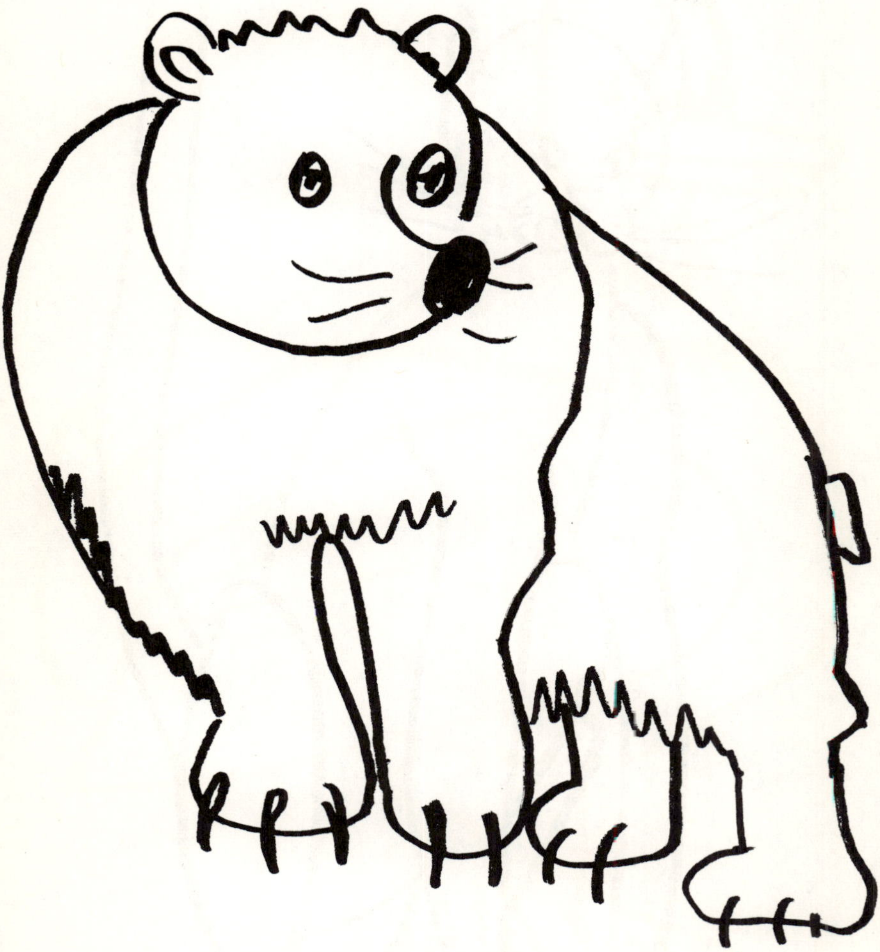

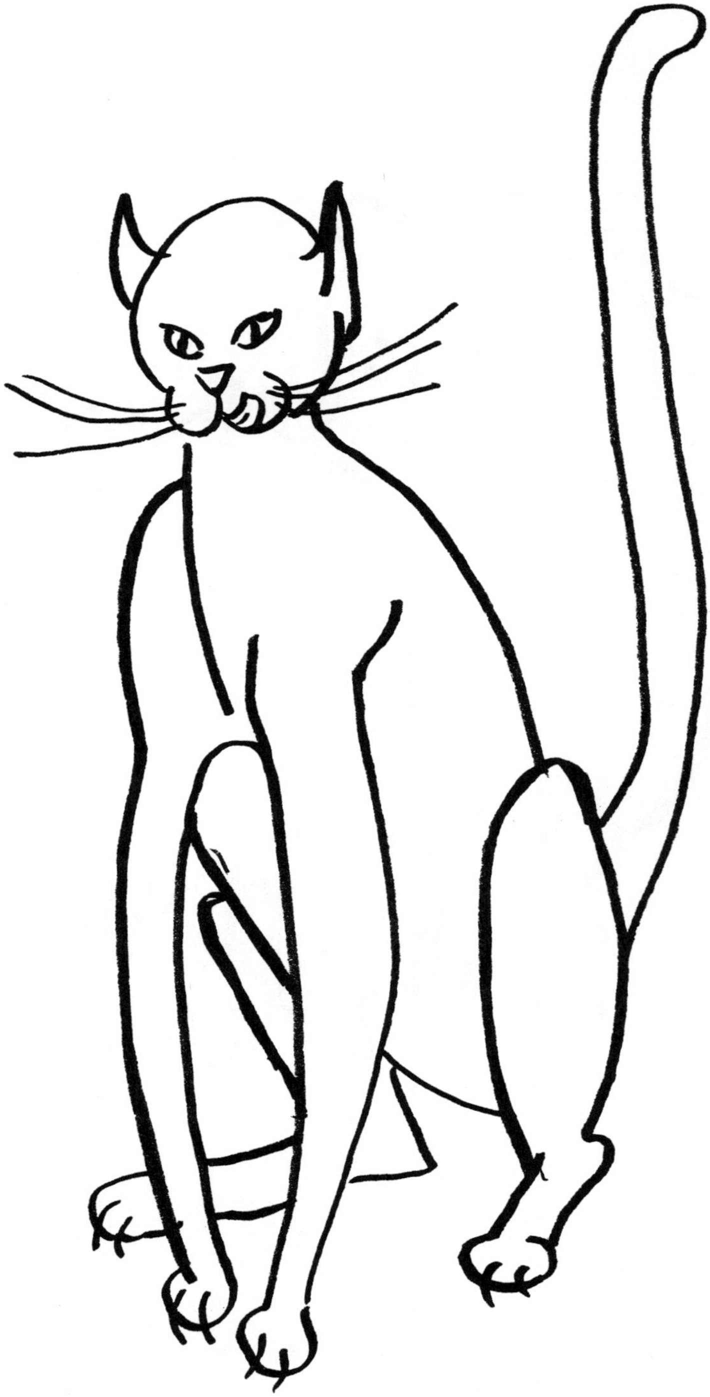

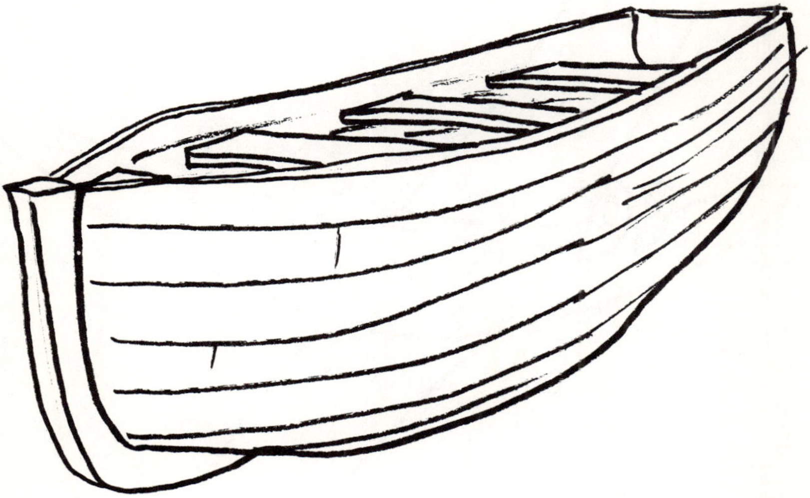

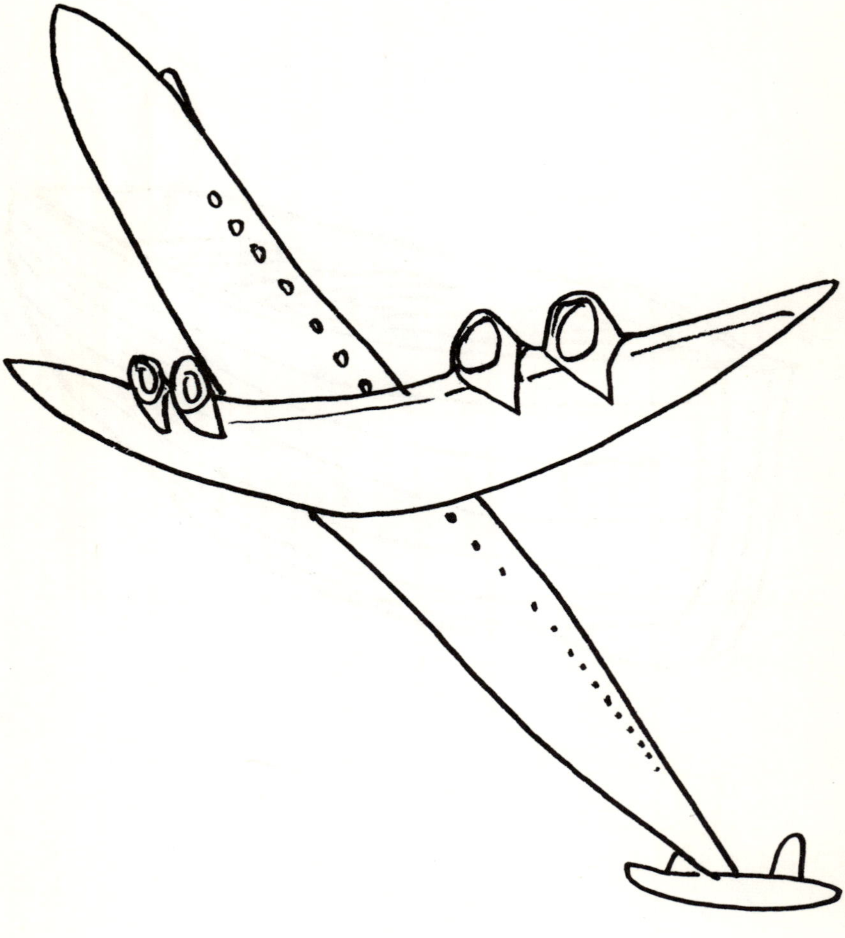

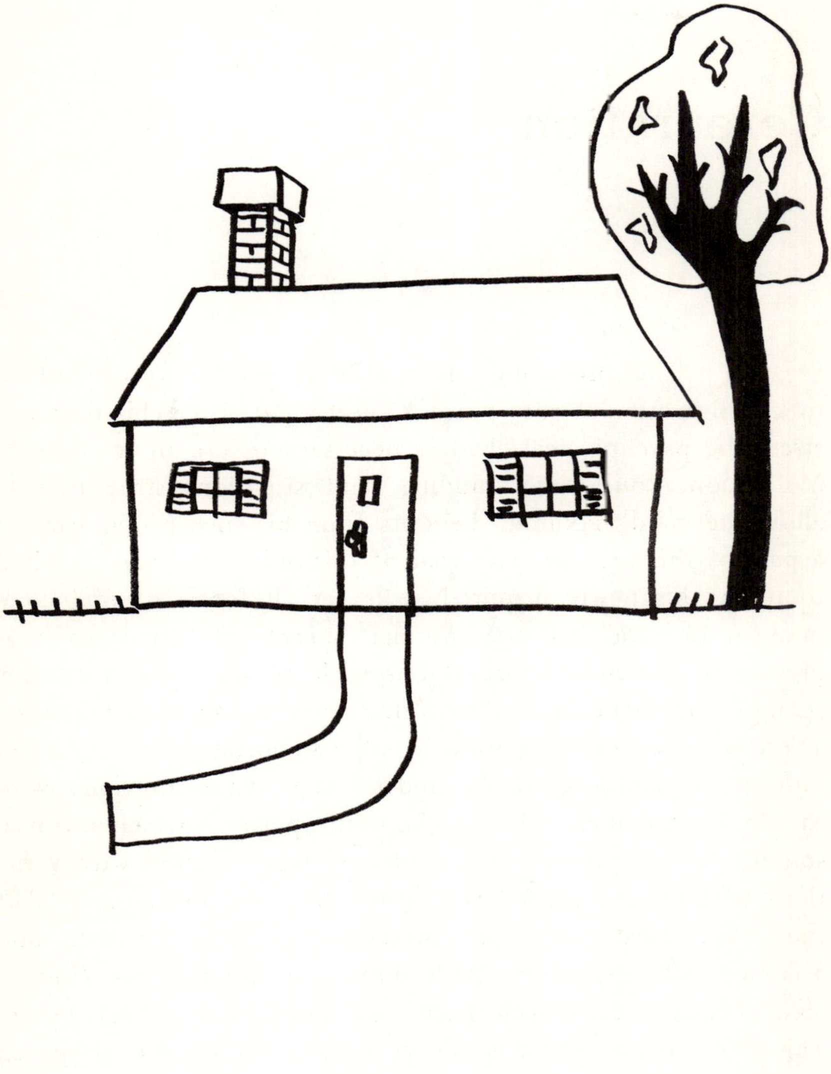

Cerebration

The preceding units utilized psychomotor controls to establish new cognitive-motor speech patterns. This unit will stress the psychological changes necessary to use these controls. Motivation, confidence building, and situations structured to allow the child maximum benefits from his speech practices are a part of this process. The goal of this unit is to train the child to utilize his newly acquired skills for all forms of oral communication, and to use normal speech in situations that previously produced stuttered speech patterns. In stuttering therapy the therapist is always dealing with the total organism. There is no one unit considered more important than any other unit in the Kopp approach, and no one area of previous work should be excluded. The psychomotor patterns which involved sounds, words, phrases, and sentences were uttered with variations of loudness, pitch levels, voice qualities, and alteration of the articulatory tract for correct range, rate, strength, and accuracy of movements. With these new controls the child is able to control the speech mechanism to produce normal speech. This controllable action is always a cause for significant speech difference.

The child must be so well trained in the use of the newly acquired and practiced controls that he can adjust to the requirements of any speaking situation automatically and with ease.

In stuttering therapy, it is useless to try to talk the stutterer out of his difficulty; he must learn good speech habits to eliminate all vestiges of his prior disorder. Therefore, the organism must be involved with direct personal experience in speaking situations that will expose the student under favorable conditions. Thus, an unpleasant feeling toward speaking can be displaced with a positive feeling. In the use of these controls motivation is central.

The following is a suggested list of structured activities designed to provide successful experience in speaking. The therapist should:

1) Construct a "tape loop" for periods of three to five seconds' playing time. Record a complete sentence and play it back so that the child can hear his good speech.
2) Use the above approach and invite the parents or other students, if in group therapy, to listen.
3) Let the child make his own recording and play it back for a short period.
4) Provide for reading experiences using object pictures, colors, phrases, and short sentences, depending upon the child's age.
5) Read the child a story and have him retell it to the therapist, the parent, or another student.
6) Ask the child to relate an experience that occurred at home, at school, at a store, or on a trip.
7) Take the student to a familiar setting, such as another classroom, and have him give a prearranged talk, for a very short duration, to the teacher or therapist. (Members of the speech clinic staff have been used often in this structured treatment.)
8) Have the child stand and recite poems. Call in others to listen, as soon as you feel the added pressure is appropriate.
9) Use a practice telephone, such as the Tele-Trainer of the Bell Telephone Company, and practice various messages, as well as telephone manners.
10) Use the telephone to have the student call a parent or friend.
11) Arrange with teachers for the student to recite daily in class, if possible. The student can either volunteer or be called upon to recite. In any event the student should be well prepared for the experience.
12) Put on skits or plays and let the child choose the character he wishes to portray. Initially, the plays should be about animals.
13) Establish a club with the members of the speech class and arrange for the trainee to be a club officer.

14) Send the child on errands within the building. Give an oral message and check to make certain no substitutions are used.
15) Arrange for the child to bring a friend to a therapy session. Have the child explain to his friend what he has been doing in therapy.
16) Arrange for the presentation of short classroom reports. Let the child say anything he wishes about the subject.
17) Help the child seek out difficult situations and overcome them.
18) Train the child to use effortless and fearless speech in all speaking situations.
19) Request that the child speak often, but not monopolize the conversation.
20) It is very important for the speaker not to place emphasis upon the auditory tract for feedback purposes. To do so places the individual in the role of a self-listener and creates a word-by-word analysis of the oral output.
21) The therapist should have no fears of a relapse. The student frequently experiences relapses in the development of new non-stuttering neuromuscular speech patterns. In general, the relapse is temporary, and the speech seldom reaches patterns displayed before therapy. The student must be prepared for this breakdown, and it must be treated with confidence by the therapist. It is not unusual to note relapses when the student fails to adhere to the strict regimen of practice, which is absolutely essential in establishing the new psychomotor patterns as listed under therapy.

In conclusion, published research reports on stuttering estimate that there are more than a million stutterers in the United States. At a point in their lives a rational method of therapy could have removed this barrier to communication and personality development. However, most of the research on this disorder has been upon causative factors, rather than therapeutic measures. Normal speech, human knowledge, and human powers meet in one; where the course is not known, the effect cannot be produced. Nature, to be commanded, must be obeyed; and that which in contemplation is as the cause is in operation the rule.

In speech science and pathology, the contemplated course is emotional instability; and the operation, by rule, is some form of mental catharsis in the form of directed, nondirected, or mis directed counseling.

The profession of speech therapy is dependent upon satisfactory therapeutic procedures. In the area of stuttering, there has been an obvious lack of effective methodology, especially methods that can be used successfully in either individual or group sessions.

The Kopp Method of therapy will meet the needs of any stuttering problem, if the child is properly motivated and trained to use his new skills.

Notes

1. Charles VanRiper, *Speech Correction Principles and Methods* (3rd ed.; Englewood Cliffs, N.J., 1963), p. 34.
2. Victor Lowenfeld, *Creative and Mental Growth* (New York, 1963), p. 477.
3. G. Klingbeil, "The Historical Background of the Modern Speech Clinic," *Journal of Speech Disorders,* IV (June 1939), 115-32.
4. *Stuttering: A Symposium,* ed. Jon Eisenson (New York, 1958).
5. This method is spelled out in detail in Elise Hahn's text entitled *Significant Theories and Therapy of Stuttering* (Stanford, 1958).
6. Speech Foundation of America, *Stuttering and Its Prevention* (Memphis, 1962), p. 152.
7. Hariet Kopp, *Some Functional Applications of Basic Phonetic Principles* (Ann Arbor, 1960), p. 45.
8. For a complete analysis of the breathing process in speech, see R. H. Stetson, *Motor Phonetics* (2nd ed.; Amsterdam, 1951).
9. George Kopp, *Syllabus for Speech Correction* (Ann Arbor, 1946).
10. George Kopp, p. 83.

11. Ralph Potter, George Kopp, and Harriet Green, *Visible Speech* (New York, 1947).
12. George Kopp, Harriet Kopp, and Angelo Angelocci, *Visible Speech Manual* (Detroit, 1961).
13. S. S. Stevens, *Handbook of Experimental Psychology* (New York, 1962), p. 540.
14. Stetson, p. 178.
15. Burleigh Shibles, "How Many Words Does a First Grade Child Know?," *The Elementary English Journal,* XLI (January 1959), pp. 42-47; C. H. Voelker, "One Thousand Most Frequently Used Words," *Quarterly Journal of Speech,* XXVI (1947), pp. 189-97; Edward Dolch, *The 2000 Commonest Words for Spelling* (Champaign, Ill., 1955); Leonard Bloomfield and Clarence L. Barnhart, *Let's Read: A Linguistic Approach* (Detroit, 1961).

Appendix: Practice Word List

A

a
able
aboard
about
above
absence
absent
accident
account
ache
across
act
acting
action
active
actual
add
addition
address
adjust
admire
adventure
advise
afar
afraid
Africa
after
afternoon
afterward
again
against
age
agent
ago
agree
ah
ahead
aid
ail
aim
air
airfield
airplane
airport
airship
airsick
aisle
alarm
alas
Alaska
alike
alive
all
alley
allow
almond
almost
alone
along
aloud
already
also
although
always
am
America
among
amount
an
ancient
and
angel
anger
angry
animal
ankle
another
answer
ant
anxious
any
anybody
anyhow
anyone
anything
anyway
anywhere
apart
apartment
apiece
appear
apple
apricot
April
apron
apt
are

arithmetic
arm
armful
arms
army
around
arrange
arrangement
arrest
arrive
arrow
art
as
ashamed
ashes
Asia
aside
ask
asleep
at
ate
athlete
Atlantic
atom
attack
attend
attention
attic
August
aunt
auto
automobile
autumn
avenue
awake
awaken
away
awful
awhile
awl
ax

B

baby
back
backbone
background
backward
bacon
bad
badge
badly
bag
bail
bake
baker
ball
balloon
ban
banana
band
bandage
bandstand
bang
banjo
bank
banker
banner
bar
barber
bare
bargain
bark
barn
barnyard
barrel
base
baseball
basement
bask
basket
basketball
bass
bat
batch
bath
bathe
bathroom
bathtub
batter
battle
bawl
bay
be
beach
bead
beak
bean
bear
beard
beast
beat
beating
beautiful
beauty
beaver
became

because
become
bed
bedroom
beds
bedtime
bee
beech
beechnut
beef
beefsteak
been
beer
beet
before
beg
began
beggar
begged
begin
begun
behave
behavior
behind
behold
being
believe
bell
bellow
belong
below
belt
bench
bend
beneath
benefit
bent
berry
beside
best
bet
better
between
Bible
bicycle
bid
big
bigger
biggest
bike
bilk
bill
billboard
bind
birch
bird
birth
birthday
biscuit
bit
bite
bitten
bitter
blab
black
blackberry
blackbird
blackness
blacksmith
blade
blame
blank
blanket
blast
blaze
bleach
bleak
bleat
bled
bleed
blend
bless
blessing
blew
blimp
blind
blindfold
blink
bliss
blister
blob
block
blonde
blood
bloom
blot
blotch
blouse
blow
blown
blue
blueberry
bluebird
bluejay
bluff
blush
boar
board

boast
boat
bobcat
body
boil
bold
bond
bone
bonfire
bonnet
book
boom
boon
boor
boost
boot
booth
border
bore
born
borrow
boss
both
bother
bottle
bottom
bought
bounce
bound
bout
bow
bowl
box
boxcar
boxer
boxes
boy
brace
bracelet
brad
brag
brain
brake
bran
branch
brand
brass
brat
brave
brawl
breach
bread
break
breakfast
breaks
breast
breath
breathe
breed
breeze
bribe
brick
bride
bridge
brief
bright
brim
bring
brink
brittle
broad
broadcast
broil
broke
broken
brood
brook
broom
broth
brother
brought
brow
brown
brush
bubble
buck
bucket
buckle
bud
budge
buffalo
bug
buggy
build
building
built
bulb
bulge
bulk
bull
bullet
bulletin
bum
bump
bumped
bumps
bun
bunch

bundle
bunk
bunny
burden
burn
burnt
burr
burst
bury
bus
bush
bushel
business
bust
bustle
busy
but
butcher
butt
butter
butterfly
button
buy
buzz
by
bye

C

cab
cabbage
cabin
cabinet
cable
cackle
cage
cake
calf
California
call
calm
calves
came
camel
camera
camp
campfire
can
canal
canary
candle
candy
cane
caned
caning
cannon
cannot
canoe
canvas
canyon
cap
cape
capital
captain
car
carbon
card
care
careful
careless
carp
carpenter
carpet
carriage
carrot
carry
cart
carve
case
cash
cast
castle
cat
catalog
catch
catcher
catching
catfish
cats
cattle
caught
cause
cave
caw
cedar
ceiling
celebrate
cellar
cells
cent
center
central
century
cereal
certain
chain
chair

chairman
chalk
champ
champion
chance
change
chap
chapter
character
charge
charm
chart
chase
chat
chatter
cheap
cheat
check
cheek
cheer
cheerful
cheese
cherry
chess
chest
chew
Chicago
chick
chicken
chief
child
children
chill
chime
chimney
chin
china
chip
chipmunk
chirp
chocolate
choice
choke
choose
chop
chore
chose
Christmas
chuck
chum
chump
church
churn
cinder
circle
circus
cities
citizen
city
claim
clam
clamp
clan
clang
clank
clap
clash
clasp
class
classroom
clatter
claw
clay
clean
clear
clearly
cleat
cleft
clerk
clever
click
cliff
climb
clinch
cling
clip
cloak
clock
clod
clog
close
clot
cloth
clothes
clothing
cloud
cloudy
clover
clown
club
cluck
clump
clung
clutch
coach
coal
coarse
coast

coat
coax
cob
cobweb
cock
cockroach
cocoa
cocoon
cod
codfish
coffee
coffeepot
cog
coil
cold
collar
college
colony
color
Colorado
colt
Columbia
column
comb
come
comfort
comic
coming
command
commercial
common
community
companion
company
compare
complain
complete
conduct
conductor
cone
confess
connect
consent
consider
constitution
contain
content
contest
continue
contrary
control
convenience
convenient
cook
cookie
cool
cooler
coolest
coop
cop
copied
copper
copy
cord
cordial
core
cork
corn
corner
correct
correctly
costly
costume
cot
cots
cottage
cotton
couch
cough
could
couldn't
count
counter
country
county
couple
courage
course
court
cousin
cover
cow
coward
cowboy
cows
cowshed
coy
cozy
crab
crack
cracker
crackle
cradle
crag
cram
cramp
cranberry
crane

crash
crate
crawl
crayon
crazy
cream
crease
creative
creed
crept
crest
crew
crib
cricket
cried
crime
crimp
cripple
croak
crock
crooked
croon
crop
cross
crotch
crouch
crow
crowd
crown
cruel
crumb
crumple
crunch
crush
crust
crutch
cry
crying
cub
cud
cuff
cull
cunning
cup
cupboard
cupful
cur
curdle
cure
curious
curl
curse
curtain
curve
cushion
custard
customer
cut
cute
cuts
cutting

D

dab
dad
daddy
dad's
daily
dairy
daisies
daisy
dam
damage
dame
damp
dance
dancer
dandelion
dandy
danger
dangerous
dangle
dare
dark
darkness
darling
darn
dart
dash
date
daughter
dawn
day
daybreak
daytime
dazzle
dead
deaf
deal
dealer
dealt
dean
dear
dearest
death
debt

deceive
December
decide
decision
deck
declare
deed
deem
deep
deeper
deer
defeat
defend
defense
definite
delicate
delight
deliver
dell
den
dent
dentist
deny
depart
department
deposit
depot
depth
describe
desert
deserve
design
desk
destroy
detective
develop

devil
dew
diamond
did
didn't
die
died
difference
different
difficult
dig
digging
dill
dim
dime
dimple
din
dine
dined
ding
ding-dong
dinner
dip
dipper
dips
direct
direction
dirt
dirty
disappear
discount
discover
discuss
disease
dish
dishes

dishpan
dishrag
disk
dislike
dismiss
display
distance
ditch
dive
divide
division
dizzy
do
dock
doctor
dodge
does
doesn't
dog
doll
dollar
dolly
done
donkey
don't
doom
door
doorbell
doorknob
doorstep
dot
dots
double
dough
doughnut
dove

down
downstairs
downtown
dozen
drab
drain
drank
drape
draw
drawer
drawing
dray
dread
dreadful
dream
drench
dress
dresser
drew
dried
dries
drift
drill
drink
drinking
drip
drive
driver
drizzle
drool
droop
drop
drove
drown
drowsy
drub
drudge
drug
drum
drunk
dry
drying
dub
duck
duckling
duct
dud
due
duel
dug
duke
dull
dumb
dump
dun
dung
during
dusk
dust
dusty
Dutch
duty
dwarf
dwell
dye
dyed
dyeing
dyes
dying

E

each
eager
eagle
ear
early
earmuff
earn
earnest
ears
earth
easier
easiest
easily
east
Easter
eastern
easy
eat
eaten
eating
ebb
edge
education
egg
eggshell
eight
eighteen
eighth
eighty
either
elbow
elect
election
elephant

eleven
elf
ell
elm
else
elsewhere
employ
empty
end
ending
enemy
engage
engine
engineer
England
English
enjoy
enough
enter
entertain
entire
entirely
entrance
envelope
equal
erase
eraser
errand
errors
escape
etch
Eve
even
evening
event
ever
every
everybody
everyday
everyone
everything
everywhere
evil
exact
examination
examine
example
except
exchange
exciting
excuse
existence
expect
expense
expensive
explain
extra
eye
eyebrow

F

face
fact
factory
facts
fade
fail
faint
fair
fairy
faith
fall
fallen
false
familiar
family
famous
fan
far
fare
farm
farmer
farther
fashion
fast
fasten
fat
fate
father
fatter
fault
favor
favorite
fawn
fear
fearful
feat
feather
feature
February
fed
fee
feed
feel
feet
fell

fellow
felt
fence
fern
fever
few
fib
fidget
field
fierce
fifteen
fifth
fifty
fig
fight
figure
file
fill
film
fin
final
financial
find
fine
finger
finish
fir
fire
firecracker
fireman
firm
first
fish
fishing
fist
fit
five
fix
flag
flail
flake
flame
flank
flap
flash
flashlight
flat
flea
fled
flee
fleece
fleet
flesh
flew
flicks
flies
flight
fling
flip
flip-flop
flit
float
flock
flog
flood
floor
flop
flour
flow
flower
flown
fluff
flung
flunk
flurry
flush
flutter
fly
flying
foam
foe
fog
foggy
foil
fold
folks
follow
fond
food
fool
foolish
foot
football
for
forbid
forbidden
force
ford
forehead
foreign
forenoon
forest
forgave
forget
forgive
forgot
fork
form

formed
former
forms
fort
forth
fortunate
fortune
forward
fought
foul
found
fountain
four
fourteen
fowl
fox
frame
France
frank
freak
free
freed
freedom
freeze
freight
French
frequent
fresh
fret
Friday
fried
friend
friendly
friendship
fries
fright

frighten
frill
fringe
frog
from
front
frost
froth
frown
froze
frozen
fruit
fry
frying
fudge
fuel
full
fully
fumble
fun
fund
funny
fur
furious
furnish
furniture
furry
furs
fuss
fussy
future
fuzz
fuzzy

G

gab
gadget
gag
gain
gal
gale
gallon
game
gang
gap
garage
garbage
garden
garment
gas
gash
gasoline
gate
gather
gauze
gave
gay
gaze
gear
geese
gem
general
generous
gentle
gentleman
geography
German
get
getting

ghost
giant
gift
gill
gilt
girl
give
given
giver
glad
gladly
glance
glass
gleam
glee
glen
glib
glide
glimmer
glimpse
glitter
globe
glory
glove
glow
glue
glum
gnash
gnat
gnaw
go
good
goal
goat
gob
gobble
God
godmother
goes
going
gold
golden
golf
gone
good
good-bye
good news
goods
goof
goose
gooseberry
gosh
got
gotten
government
governor
gown
grab
grabbed
gracious
grade
grades
gradual
graduate
graduation
grain
gram
grand
grandchild
grandfather
grandmother
grandpa
grandson
grandstand
granite
grant
grass
grasshopper
grate
grave
gravel
gravy
gray
great
greatest
Greece
greed
greedy
green
greet
grew
grey
grid
grief
grieve
grill
grim
grin
grind
grip
gristle
grit
groan
grocery
groom
groove
grouch
ground

group
grouse
grow
growl
grown
growth
grub
grudge
gruel
gruff
grumble
grumbling
grunt
guarantee
guard
guardian
guess
guest
guide
guilt
guilty
gulch
gulf
gull
gum
gumdrops
gun
gunpowder
guns
gunsmith
gush
gust
gut
guy
gymnasium

H

habit
had
hadn't
hag
hail
hair
haircut
hairpin
half
hall
halt
halter
halves
ham
hammer
hammock
hand
handbag
handcuff
handful
handkerchief
handle
handwriting
hang
happen
happier
happiest
happiness
happy
harbor
hard
hardly
hardware
hare
hark
harm
harness
harp
harvest
has
hash
hasn't
haste
hasten
hat
hatch
hatchet
hate
haunch
have
haven't
having
hawk
hay
haystack
he
head
headache
heal
health
healthy
heap
hear
heard
hearing
heart
hearth
heat
heater
heaven

heavy
hedge
heed
heel
heels
height
held
hell
he'll
hello
helm
helmet
help
helper
helpful
hem
hemp
hen
hence
her
herd
here
hero
hers
herself
he's
hesitate
hey
hid
hidden
hide
high
higher
highness
highway
hike
hill
hilltop
hilly
hilt
him
himself
hinge
hint
hip
hire
his
hiss
history
hit
hitch
hither
hits
hitter
hive
ho
hoax
hob
hoe
hoeing
hoes
hog
hoist
hold
holder
hole
holiday
hollow
holly
holy
home
homestead
honest
honesty
honey
honk
honor
hood
hoof
hook
hoop
hoot
hop
hope
hopeful
hopeless
horn
horrible
horrid
horse
horseback
hose
hospital
host
hot
hotel
hound
hour
house
houses
how
however
howl
hub
huff
hug
huge
hulk

hull
hum
human
hump
hundred
hung
hunger
hungry
hunk
hunt
hunted
hunter
hurdle
hurry
hurt
husband
hush
husk
hustle
hut
hutch
huts
hymn
hyphen

I

I
ice
icebox
ice cream
icy
idea
idle
if
igloo
ill
I'll
I'm
imagine
imp
impatient
important
impossible
improve
improvement
in
inch
increase
indeed
India
Indian
Indiana
individual
indoor
ink
inn
inquire
insect
inside
insist
instant
instead
instruct
insult
insurance
intend
interest
interested
interesting
into
invent
investigate
invite
iron
is
island
isle
isn't
issue
it
Italian
itch
its
it's
itself
I've
ivory
ivy

J

jab
Jack Frost
jacket
jacknife
jag
jail
jam
January
jar
jaunt
jaw
jay
jazz
jealous

jelly
jerk
Jesus
jet
jets
jiffy
jig
jilt
jingle
jinx
job
jog
join
joining
joint
joke
jolly
jot
jowl
joy
joyful
judge
judgment
jug
juggle
juice
juicy
July
jump
jumped
June
junior
junk
junket
just
jut

K

keel
keen
keep
keg
kep
ketch
kettle
key
kick
kid
kill
killed
kilt
kin
kind
kindle
kindness
king
kingdom
kiss
kissed
kisses
kitchen
kite
kitten
kitty
knack
knee
kneel
knelt
knew
knife
knight
knit
knives
knob
knock
knot
know
known

L

lab
label
labor
lace
lack
lad
ladder
ladies
lady
lag
laid
lain
lair
lake
lakes
lamb
lame
lamp
lance
land
landed
lane
language
lank
lantern
lap

lapse
lard
large
lark
lash
last
latch
late
later
latest
lathe
lather
laugh
launch
law
lawn
laws
lawyer
lax
lay
layer
lazy
lea
lead
leader
leaf
leak
lean
leap
learn
lease
leash
least
leather
leave
leaves

lecture
led
ledge
leech
leek
left
leg
lemon
lemonade
lend
length
leopard
less
lesson
lest
let
letter
lettuce
level
library
lice
lick
lid
lie
lied
life
lifeguard
lift
light
lightning
like
lilt
lily
lima beans
limb
limber

lime
limp
line
linen
link
lint
lion
lioness
lip
liquid
lisp
list
listen
lit
literature
little
live
lived
liver
lives
living
lizard
load
loaf
loam
loan
loaves
lob
local
locate
lock
locker
locking
lodge
loft
log

lone
lonely
long
longer
longest
look
loom
loon
loop
loose
loot
lop
lope
lord
lose
loser
loss
lost
lot
loud
lounge
louse
lout
love
lovely
luck
lucky
lug
lull
lumber
lumps
lunch
lung
lying

M

machine
machinery
mad
made
magazine
magic
maid
mail
mailbox
mailman
main
maintain
major
make
maker
male
malt
malted milk
mama
man
manager
mane
manger
manner
manufacture
many
map
maple
mar
marble
March
mare
mark
market
marriage
married
marry
marsh
mask
mass
mast
master
mat
match
mate
material
matter
mattress
May
maybe
mayor
me
meadow
meal
mean
meaning
meant
meantime
measure
meat
medicine
meek
meet
meeting
mellow
melt
member
men
mend
mention

meow
mere
merit
merry
mesh
mess
message
messenger
met
metal
method
mew
mice
Michigan
mid
middle
midget
midnight
miff
might
mighty
mild
mile
milk
milkmaid
milkman
mill
miller
million
mind
minded
mine
mineral
mink
mint
minute
mirror
mischief
miss
misspell
mist
mistake
mistaken
mitt
mitten
mix
mixing
mixture
moan
moat
mob
mock
model
moist
mold
mole
moment
Monday
money
monkey
month
monthly
moo
mood
moon
moonbeam
moonlight
moonshine
moor
moose
moot
mop
mope
mops
more
moreover
morning
moss
most
mostly
moth
mother
motion
motor
mound
mount
mountain
mourn
mouse
mouth
move
movement
movie
mow
much
muck
mud
muddy
muff
mug
mulch
mule
mull
mum
mumble
munch
murder
muscle

mush
music
musk
muss
must
mustache
mustard
mutt
mutter
mutton
mutual
my
myself
mystery

N

nab
nag
nail
name
named
names
nap
napkin
narrow
nasty
nation
national
native
natural
naughty
navy
nay
near
nearby
nearly
neat
necessary
neck
necktie
need
needle
needn't
neglect
Negro
neighbor
neighborhood
neither
nest
nests
net
nettle
never
new
news
newspaper
New York
next
nib
nibble
nice
nicely
nickel
niece
night
nightgown
nine
nineteen
ninety
ninth
nip
no
noble
nobody
nod
noise
noisy
none
noodle
nook
noon
noose
nor
normal
north
northern
nose
not
notch
note
nothing
notice
notion
November
now
nowhere
nub
nudge
nuisance
null
numb
number
numeral
numerous
nun
nurse

nut
nuts

O

oaf
oar
oars
oath
oatmeal
oats
oatseed
obedient
obey
object
occasion
occasionally
ocean
o'clock
October
odd
of
off
offer
office
officer
official
often
oh
oil
old
older
olive
on
once
one
onion
only
onto
onward
open
operate
opposite
or
orange
orchard
order
ore
organ
orphan
other
otherwise
ouch
ought
ounce
our
ourselves
out
outdoors
outfit
outlaw
outline
outside
oven
over
overalls
overcoat
overhead
overnight
overturn
owe
owl
own
owner
ox
oxen
oyster

P

pace
pack
package
pact
pad
page
paid
pail
pain
painful
paint
paintbrush
painter
painting
pair
pal
palace
pale
palm
pan
pancake
pane
panel
panes
pang
pans

pants
pap
papa
paper
parade
paragraph
pardon
parent
parents
park
parlor
part
partly
partner
partnership
party
pass
passage
passenger
past
paste
pasting
pasture
pat
patch
path
patient
pattern
paunch
pave
pawn
pay
pea
peace
peaceful
peach
peak
peal
peanut
pear
pearl
peat
peck
peculiar
pedal
peek
peel
peep
peer
peeve
peg
pelt
pep
pencil
pend
pennies
Pennsylvania
penny
pent
people
pep
pepper
perch
perfect
perfume
perhaps
period
person
pet
petal
pew
Philadelphia
phone
photo
photograph
physical
physician
piano
pick
pickle
pickup
picnic
picture
pie
piece
pig
pigeon
pigpen
pile
pill
pillow
pin
pinch
pine
ping
pink
pint
pip
pipe
pioneer
pistol
pit
pitch
pitcher
pitching
pity
place
plain

plan
plane
planing
plank
plant
plat
plate
platform
platter
play
played
player
playground
playmate
plaything
pleasant
please
pleasure
plenty
plod
plot
plow
pluck
plug
plum
plump
plus
plush
poach
pock
pocket
pod
poem
point
pointer
poison
poke
pole
police
policeman
polish
polite
pond
pony
poof
pool
poor
pop
popcorn
pope
popgun
popular
population
porch
pork
port
pose
possible
post
postage
postal
pot
potato
pots
pouch
pounce
pound
pour
powder
power
powerful
practice
praise
prank
pray
prayer
preach
preacher
precious
prep
prepare
present
president
press
pretty
prevent
prey
price
pride
priest
prince
princess
principal
print
prison
prisoner
prize
probably
problem
prod
product
program
prom
promise
prompt
proof
prop
proper

protect
proud
prove
prowl
prune
pudding
puff
pug
pull
pulp
pulse
pump
pumpkin
pun
punch
punish
punk
punt
puny
pupil
puppy
pure
purple
purpose
purr
purse
pus
push
pussy
put
puzzle

Q

quack
quail
quaint
quake
quality
quantity
quarrel
quart
quarter
queer
quell
quench
quest
question
quick
quickly
quiet
quill
quilt
quip
quit
quite
quiz

R

rabbit
race
rack
radio
radish
raft
rag
rage
raid
rail
railroad
railway
rain
rainbow
rainy
raise
raisin
rake
raked
raking
ram
ramble
ramp
ran
ranch
rang
range
ranger
rank
rant
rap
rapid
rapped
rare
rash
rat
rate
rather
rattle
rattler
rave
raw
ray
razor
reach
reaching

read
reading
ready
real
really
rear
reason
receive
recognize
record
red
reduce
reek
reel
refuse
regular
reign
reindeer
reins
relative
remember
remove
rent
repair
repeat
report
request
require
respect
rest
result
return
review
reward
rib
ribbon
rice
rick
rid
ride
ridge
rift
rig
right
rim
ring
rink
rinse
rip
ripe
riper
ripple
rise
risk
river
roach
road
roam
roan
roar
roast
rob
robber
robin
rock
rocket
rod
rode
roll
rolling
romp
roof
room
rooster
root
rope
rose
rot
rotten
rouge
rough
round
rout
route
rove
row
rowboat
royal
rub
rubber
rubbish
rudder
rude
ruff
rug
ruin
rule
ruler
rum
rumble
rump
run
rung
runner
running
runt
rush
Russia

rust
rusty
rut
rye

S

sack
sad
sadness
safe
safest
safety
sag
sage
said
sail
sailboat
sailor
saint
sake
salad
salary
sale
salesman
salt
same
sample
sand
sandbox
sandwich
sandy
sang
sank
Santa Claus
sap
sash
sat
satellite
satin
satisfactory
Saturday
saucer
sausage
savage
save
saver
saves
saw
say
scab
scale
scamp
scan
scar
scarce
scare
scared
scarf
scat
scatter
scene
scent
schedule
scheme
school
schoolbag
schoolhouse
schoolmaster
schoolroom
schoolteacher
science
scissors
scold
scoop
scoot
scooter
scorch
score
scorn
scotch
scour
scout
scow
scowl
scram
scramble
scrap
scrape
scratch
scrawl
screech
screen
screw
script
scrub
scuff
scum
sea
seal
seam
search
season
seat
second
secret
secretary

see
seed
seeing
seek
seem
seen
seep
seesaw
seize
seldom
self
sell
semester
send
senior
sense
sent
sentence
separate
September
serious
servant
serve
service
set
settle
settlement
settler
seven
seventh
seventy
several
severe
sew
shack
shad
shade
shadow
shady
shaft
shake
shall
shame
shank
shape
share
shark
sharp
sharpen
shatter
shave
shaver
shaving
shawl
she
sheaf
sheath
shed
sheep
sheer
sheet
shelf
shell
shelter
shelve
shepherd
shield
shift
shine
shingle
ship
shirk
shirt
shiver
shock
shoe
shoo
shook
shoot
shooter
shop
shopper
shopping
shore
short
shot
shotgun
should
shoulder
shouldn't
shout
shove
shovel
show
shower
shown
shred
shrill
shrimp
shrink
shrub
shrug
shrunk
shuck
shudder
shun
shunt
shut

shutter
shy
sick
sickness
side
sidewalk
siding
sieve
sift
sigh
sight
sign
signal
signature
silence
silent
silk
sill
silly
silt
silver
silverware
simmer
simple
sin
since
sincerely
sing
singer
singing
single
sink
sinker
sip
sir
sister
sit
sitting
situation
six
sixteen
sixteenth
sixth
sixty
size
sizzle
skate
skater
skating
sketch
ski
skid
skies
skiff
skill
skim
skimp
skin
skip
skirt
skit
skull
skunk
sky
slab
slack
slag
slam
slammed
slang
slap
slash
slat
slaughter
slave
slay
sled
sleep
sleepy
sleet
sleeve
sleigh
slept
slice
slick
slid
slide
slight
slim
slime
slimy
slip
slipped
slipper
slippery
slit
sliver
sloop
slope
slosh
slot
slouch
slow
slowly
slug
slum
slumber
slump

slung
slush
sly
smack
small
smart
smear
smell
smelled
smelt
smile
smiling
smoke
smooth
smudge
smug
snack
snag
snail
snake
snap
snatch
sneak
sneeze
snicker
sniff
snip
snoop
snore
snout
snow
snowfall
snowflake
snowy
snub
snuff
snuggle
so
soak
soap
soar
sob
social
sock
sod
soda
sofa
soft
softly
soil
sold
soldier
sole
solid
solve
some
somebody
somehow
someone
something
sometime
somewhat
somewhere
son
song
soon
sooner
soot
sop
sore
sorrow
sorry
sort
sought
soul
sound
sounds
soup
sour
south
southern
sow
soy
space
spade
Spain
span
spank
spare
spark
sparkle
sparrow
spat
speak
speaker
spear
special
sped
speed
spell
spelling
spend
spent
spice
spider
spike
spill
spilt

spin
spinach
spirit
spit
spite
splash
splendid
splint
split
spoil
spoke
spoken
spook
spool
spoon
sport
spot
spout
sprain
sprawl
spray
spread
spree
spring
sprinkle
sprinkler
sprout
spruce
sprung
spud
spun
spurn
spy
squall
square
squash
squat
squawk
squeak
squeal
squeeze
squelch
squib
squid
squint
squirm
squirrel
squirt
stab
stable
stack
stag
stage
stain
stair
stale
stall
stamp
stand
standard
star
starch
stare
start
starve
state
station
statue
stay
staying
stead
steal
steam
steamboat
steamer
steamship
steel
steep
steer
stem
step
stepmother
stern
stew
stick
sticky
stiff
still
stillness
stir
stitch
stock
stocking
stole
stone
stood
stool
stoop
stop
stopper
stopping
store
stork
storm
stormy
story
stout
stove

straight
strain
strand
strange
stranger
strap
straw
strawberry
stray
streak
stream
street
strength
stress
stretch
strew
strict
strife
strike
string
strip
stripe
strode
stroll
strong
stronger
struck
struggle
strum
strung
stub
stuck
stud
student
studied
studies
study
stuff
stumble
stun
stung
stunt
stupid
style
styles
sub
subject
succeed
such
sudden
suddenly
suffer
sufficient
sugar
suit
sulk
sum
summer
summon
sun
sunbeam
Sunday
sunflower
sung
sunk
sunlight
sunny
sunrise
sunset
sunshine
supper
support
suppose
sure
surely
surface
surprise
surround
swallow
swamp
swan
swank
swarm
swat
sway
swear
sweat
sweater
sweep
sweet
sweetheart
sweetness
swell
swept
swift
swill
swim
swimming
swing
swish
Swiss
switch
swollen
swoon
swoop
sword
swore
sworn

swum
swung
sympathy
syrup
system

T

tab
table
tablecloth
tablespoon
tablet
tabulated
tack
tackle
tact
tag
tail
tailor
taint
take
taken
talc
tale
talk
tan
tang
tangle
tank
tap
tape
tapes
tar
tardy
target
task
taste
tastes
taught
taunt
tax
taxes
tea
teach
teacher
teak
team
tear
tease
teased
teaspoon
tee
teen
teeter
teeth
telegraph
telephone
tell
temper
temperature
temple
tempt
ten
tender
tennis
tent
terrible
test
text
than
thank
thanked
thankful
thanks
Thanksgiving
that
thaw
the
theater
their
theirs
them
themselves
then
there
therefore
these
they
they're
they've
thick
thicker
thickest
thicket
thief
thigh
thimble
thin
thing
think
thinking
thinner
third
thirst
thirsty
thirteen

thirty
this
thorn
thorough
those
though
thought
thousand
thrash
thread
threat
threaten
three
thresh
threw
thrift
thrill
throat
throne
throng
through
throughout
throw
thrown
thrush
thrust
thumb
thump
thunder
Thursday
tick
ticket
tickle
tickled
tide
tie

tied
ties
tiger
tight
tighten
tile
till
tilt
timber
time
timed
times
timing
tin
ting
tingle
tinkle
tiny
tip
tipped
tiptoe
tire
tired
title
to
toad
toadstool
toast
tobacco
today
toe
toes
tog
together
toil
toilet

token
told
tomato
tomorrow
ton
tone
tongue
tonight
too
took
tool
toot
tooth
toothbrush
toothpick
top
topple
torch
tore
torn
toss
tot
total
touch
tough
tow
toward
towel
tower
town
toy
trace
track
tract
trade
trader

trades
trading
traffic
trail
train
trait
tramp
trap
trash
travel
tray
tread
treasure
treat
tree
trees
treetop
tremble
trench
trend
trick
trickle
tricycle
tries
trill
trim
trip
troll
troop
trot
trouble
trough
trout
truck
true
truly
trump
trumpet
trunk
trust
truth
try
trying
tub
Tuesday
tug
tulip
tumble
tune
tunnel
turkey
turn
turnip
turtle
tusk
twain
twang
tweed
tweet
twelfth
twelve
twenty
twice
twig
twin
twine
twinkle
twirl
twist
two
tying
type
typed
typewriter
typing
typist

U

ugly
umbrella
unable
uncle
under
understand
understood
undress
uneasy
unfair
unfinished
unfold
unfriendly
unhappy
unhurt
union
unite
United States
unkind
unless
unpaid
until
unusual
unwilling
up
upon
upper
upset

upstairs
uptown
upwards
urge
us
use
used
useful
useless
usual
usually
utter

V

vacation
vain
valentine
valley
valuable
vamp
van
vase
vat
veal
vegetable
vein
velvet
vend
vent
very
vest
vet
vetch
vex

victory
view
village
vine
violent
violet
visit
visitor
voice
vote
vow
voyage

W

wad
wade
waded
wading
wag
wagon
wail
waist
wait
wake
waken
walk
wall
walnut
wand
wander
want
war
ware
warm

warn
wart
was
wash
Washington
washtub
wasn't
wasp
waste
watch
watchman
water
watermelon
waterproof
wave
wax
way
we
weak
weaken
weakness
wealth
wean
weapon
wear
weary
weather
weave
web
wed
wedding
wedge
Wednesday
wee
weed
weeded

week
weekend
weep
weigh
weight
welcome
weld
well
we'll
welt
went
wept
were
weren't
west
western
wet
we've
whale
what
whatever
wheat
wheel
when
where
wherever
whether
which
while
whim
whip
whirl
whish
whisk
whiskers
whisper
whistle
white
whiz
who
whole
whom
whose
why
wick
wide
width
wife
wig
wiggle
wild
wildcat
willing
will
willow
wilt
win
winch
wind
windmill
window
windy
wine
wiggle
winner
winter
wipe
wiping
wire
wired
wiring
wisdom
wise
wiser
wisest
wish
wishbone
wished
wishes
wisp
wit
witch
with
withdraw
wither
within
without
wives
wizard
woke
wolf
woman
women
won
wonder
wonderful
won't
woo
wood
wooden
woods
wool
woolen
word
wore
work
world
worm

worn
worry
worse
worship
worst
worth
would
wouldn't
wound
wrap
wreath
wreck
wren
wrench
wring
wringer
wrist
write
writer
writing
written
wrong
wrote

Y

yam
yank
yap
yard
yarn
year
yeast
yell
yellow
yelp
yen
yes
yesterday
yet
yield
yolk
yonder
you
younger
youngster
your
yourselves
youth

Z

zero
zest
zing
zip
zipper
zoo
zoom

Elwood G. Anderson is Supervising Teacher in Speech Therapy with the Detroit Public Schools and part-time instructor of Speech Pathology at Wayne State University and associate professor at Marygrove College.

A former stutterer, Dr. Anderson overcame his disorder completely after treatment by Dr. George A. Kopp, who developed the Kopp Method. Professor Anderson worked with Dr. Kopp at the Wayne State University Speech and Hearing Clinic until Kopp's death in 1968.

The manuscript was edited by Linda Grant. The book was designed by Mary Jowski. The type face is Caledonia designed by W. A. Dwiggins and the display face is Craw Clarendon designed by Freeman Craw. The paper used is Glatfelter's P. & S. Wove and the book is bound with Columbia Mills Bayside Chambray BVC over Binders Boards. Manufactured in the United States of America.